Barbara Jo Brothers
Editor

When One Partner
Is Willing
and the Other Is Not

Pre-Publication
REVIEWS,
COMMENTARIES,
EVALUATIONS . . .

"**B**arbara Jo Brothers has assembled an engaging variety of insightful perspectives on resistance in couples therapy. The reader comes away with a range of explanations for the many ways in which the course of progress can break down, and learns how to turn these roadblocks into valuable learning experiences for the client. Not a 'one size fits all' explanation, but a sound basis for flexible, individualized assessments and treatment strategies."

Stan Taubman, DSW
Director of Managed Care
Alameda County
Behavioral Health Care Service
Berkeley, California

The Haworth Press, Inc.

The Haworth Press, Inc.

When One Partner Is Willing and the Other Is Not

When One Partner
Is Willing
and the Other Is Not

Barbara Jo Brothers
Editor

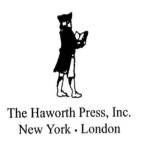

The Haworth Press, Inc.
New York · London

When One Partner Is Willing and the Other Is Not has also been published as *Journal of Couples Therapy,* Volume 7, Number 1 1997.

The development, preparation, and publication of this work has been undertaken with great care. However, the publisher, employees, editors, and agents of The Haworth Press and all imprints of The Haworth Press, Inc., including The Haworth Medical Press and Pharmaceutical Products Press, are not responsible for any errors contained herein or for consequences that may ensue from use of materials or information contained in this work. Opinions expressed by the author(s) are not necessarily those of The Haworth Press, Inc.

The Haworth Press, Inc., 10 Alice Street, Binghamton, NY 13904-1580 USA

Library of Congress Cataloging-in-Publication Data

When one partner is willing and the other is not / Barbara Jo Brothers, editor.
    p. cm.
    Includes bibliographical references and index.
    ISBN 0-7890-0038-5 (alk. paper)–ISBN 0-7890-0342-2 (pbk.)
    1. Marital psychotherapy. 2. Resistance (Psychoanalysis) 3. Communication in marriage. I. Brothers, Barbara Jo, 1940- .
RC488.5.W467 1997
616.89′ 156–dc21

                                              96-51966
                                                  CIP

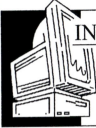

INDEXING & ABSTRACTING

Contributions to this publication are selectively indexed or abstracted in print, electronic, online, or CD-ROM version(s) of the reference tools and information services listed below. This list is current as of the copyright date of this publication. See the end of this section for additional notes.

- *Abstracts of Research in Pastoral Care & Counseling*, Loyola College, 7135 Minstrel Way, Suite 101, Columbia, MD 21045

- *CNPIEC Reference Guide: Chinese Directory of Foreign Periodicals*, P.O. Box 88, Beijing, People's Republic of China

- *Family Studies Database (online and CD/ROM)*, National Information Services Corporation, 306 East Baltimore Pike, 2nd Floor, Media, PA 19063

- *Family Violence & Sexual Assault Bulletin*, Family Violence & Sexual Assault Institute, 1121 East South East Loop 323, Suite 130, Tyler, TX 75701

- *INTERNET ACCESS (& additional networks) Bulletin Board for Libraries ("BUBL"), coverage of information resources on INTERNET, JANET, and other networks.*
  - JANET X.29: UK.AC.BATH.BUBL or 00006012101300
  - TELNET: BUBL.BATH.AC.UK or 138.38.32.45 login 'bubl'
  - Gopher: BUBL.BATH.AC.UK (138.32.32.45). Port 7070
  - World Wide Web: http: / / www.bubl.bath.ac.uk./BUBL/home.html
  - NISSWAIS: telnetniss.ac.uk (for the NISS gateway)
  The Andersonian Library, Curran Building, 101 St. James Road, Glasgow G4 ONS, Scotland

- *Mental Health Abstracts (online through DIALOG)*, IFI/Plenum Data Company, 3202 Kirkwood Highway, Wilmington, DE 19808

- *Referativnyi Zhurnal (Abstracts Journal of the Institute of Scientific Information of the Republic of Russia)*, The Institute of Scientific Information, Baltijskaja ul., 14, Moscow A-219, Republic of Russia

(continued)

- *Social Planning/Policy & Development Abstracts (SOPODA)*, Sociological Abstracts, Inc., P.O. Box 22206, San Diego, CA 92192-0206

- *Social Work Abstracts*, National Association of Social Workers, 750 First Street NW, 8th Floor, Washington, DC 20002

- *Sociological Abstracts (SA)*, Sociological Abstracts, Inc., P.O. Box 22206, San Diego, CA 92192-0206

- *Studies on Women Abstracts*, Carfax Publishing Company, P.O. Box 25, Abingdon, Oxfordshire OX14 3UE, United Kingdom

- *Violence and Abuse Abstracts: A Review of Current Literature on Interpersonal Violence (VAA)*, Sage Publications, Inc., 2455 Teller Road, Newbury Park, CA 91320

SPECIAL BIBLIOGRAPHIC NOTES

related to special journal issues (separates) and indexing/abstracting

❏ indexing/abstracting services in this list will also cover material in any "separate" that is co-published simultaneously with Haworth's special thematic journal issue or DocuSerial. Indexing/abstracting usually covers material at the article/chapter level.

❏ monographic co-editions are intended for either non-subscribers or libraries which intend to purchase a second copy for their circulating collections.

❏ monographic co-editions are reported to all jobbers/wholesalers/approval plans. The source journal is listed as the "series" to assist the prevention of duplicate purchasing in the same manner utilized for books-in-series.

❏ to facilitate user/access services all indexing/abstracting services are encouraged to utilize the co-indexing entry note indicated at the bottom of the first page of each article/chapter/contribution.

❏ this is intended to assist a library user of any reference tool (whether print, electronic, online, or CD-ROM) to locate the monographic version if the library has purchased this version but not a subscription to the source journal.

❏ individual articles/chapters in any Haworth publication are also available through the Haworth Document Delivery Services (HDDS).

When One Partner Is Willing and the Other Is Not

CONTENTS

ABOUT THE EDITOR

Barbara Jo Brothers, MSW, BCD, a Diplomate in Clinical Social Work, National Association of Social Workers, is in private practice in New Orleans. She received her BA from the University of Texas and her MSW from Tulane University, where she is currently on the faculty. She was Editor of *The Newsletter of the American Academy of Psychotherapists* from 1976 to 1985, and was Associate Editor of *Voices: The Art and Science of Psychotherapy* from 1979 to 1989. She has 30 years of experience, in both the public and private sectors, helping people to form skills that will enable them to connect emotionally. The author of numerous articles and book chapters on authenticity in human relating, she has advocated healthy, congruent communication that builds intimacy as opposed to destructive, incongruent communication which blocks intimacy. In addition to her many years of direct work with couples and families, Ms. Brothers has led numerous workshops on teaching communication in families and has also played an integral role in the development of training programs in family therapy for mental health workers throughout the Louisiana state mental health system. She is a board member of the Institute for International Connections, a non-profit organization for cross-cultural professional development focused on training and cross-cultural exchange with psychotherapists in Russia, republics once part of what used to be the Soviet Union, and other Eastern European countries.

Ways of Viewing the World

Ways of Putting Things Together to Form the Big Picture

A View of Resistance as a Blessing

Virginia Satir

EDITOR'S NOTE. The following is one of a series of lectures; Avanta Process Community Meeting III, Crested Butte, Colorado, August 1983. Transcribed and published by John Banmen (1983), this lecture had been given during the early part of a 30 day residential seminar; as always, it was accompanied by demonstrations which illustrated the points. Virginia's teaching mode was directed at the whole person, not simply the intellect. To engage both body and emotions, she would weave her lectures in among her exercises and demonstrations, over a month's time; a tapestry would form, one illustrating the other. Admittedly, there are problems with lifting, out of context, one hour or two of these summations of her many years of clinical observation. Never linear herself, Virginia understood the interactions of the world, human elements as well as non-human, as sets of nested systems. "It is not about content"; Virginia used to say, "it is all about process."

The reader must bear in mind the multiple dimensions lying beneath this single dimension of the written word–and that these pages contain principles that Virginia was taking a full month to explain.

Words in brackets are editorial additions for the sake of clarity.

[Haworth co-indexing entry note]: "Ways of Viewing the World: Ways of Putting Things Together to Form the Big Picture, A View of Resistance as a Blessing." Satir, Virginia. Co-published simultaneously in *Journal of Couples Therapy* (The Haworth Press, Inc.) Vol. 7, No. 1, 1997, pp. 1-7; and: *When One Partner Is Willing and the Other Is Not* (ed: Barbara Jo Brothers) The Haworth Press, Inc., 1997, pp. 1-7.

INTRODUCTORY COMMENTARY

Barbara Jo Brothers

Virginia's teaching on how we come to an understanding of events and why change is so difficult is very relevant to resistance in its various forms.

*Virginia understood that the explanations we have been given (and then, in turn, give ourselves) about "how things are" become the ground of the perspective from which we view the world and chart our operations within it. Therefore our attitude to change is automatically resistant: who wants the earth or where they stand to buckle and heave? We are dealing with inescapable and crucial realities: the past from which and by which our perspective is shaped; the present, which persistently and inexorably invites to fluidity or stagnating growth or decline; life or death. Movement toward either pole of these three dualities is absolutely inevitable. Movement is change. What Virginia ardently wants to encourage is choice of change on the side of fluidity–growth–life. So she first carefully explains the rather random **process** by which our perspective has been constructed. She then invites us to examine and adjust at least provisionally the geology of that small terrain; then she brings into sharp focus our rather mechanical "But." She wants us to become so conscious of our resistance that our resistance becomes, as it were, a sign above two doors:*

Different Way
The Same Way.

She wants this consciousness to be a kind of space in which we are then truly free to choose either path rather than to be helplessly determined by our past to go along the same way, i.e., maintain the status quo.

FROM VIRGINIA

Four Relevant Factors

I noticed as I went through all the people [in my years of experience]–in most all of the [major] countries in the world with all kinds of symptoms, . . . I found out that most of the things [we] used to pay attention to are absolutely irrelevant when it came to working with the person themselves.

I found there are only four things that were relevant:

1. How one defines a relationship; all that goes into pairing
2. How one defines a person: who is a person, the definition of a person
3. The explanation of an event: how did it all happen?
4. Attitude towards change

Explanation of an Event

Linear Thinking Promotes "Righteousness"

Let's look at [one] explanation of events which [says]: When something happens, of course, there is "one right answer" [about why] . . . And who do you suppose has the right [answer]? The one who is on top. And, of course, one "cause," one effect. *Linear,* o.k.? So the thinking becomes A causes B and that is all.

So now we have another theory. I am sure that many of you in your training . . . thought, "What a crock that is! It doesn't fit any of my experiences." . . . Or you meet a little boy, red-headed, age five, at six o'clock in the afternoon on Tuesday, August 14th, and he has a temper tantrum. Tuesday, August 20th, five o'clock, another six year old boy having a temper tantrum. We now have a theory. Red-headed boys, age six—age five, at six o'clock on Tuesdays will have temper tantrums and if they do not, we will figure out so they can . . . Ok. A causes B. This is linear thinking. One right way and this paves the way for righteousness. And you know if you are *right.* . . All right.

Simplistic Conclusions

A causes B, one variable, one effect. What a travesty on a human being. One cause for everything. You bite your nails, that is because your grandmother does not do what she is supposed to do. Or, in another place, you eat too much. That is because you have got Cindy for a girlfriend and she is giving you wrong support. . . . . When you catch yourself [making these simplistic kinds of conclusions], let it be a cosmic joke and laugh and forget about it.

An Example

Now I will tell you this story and if it were not so true to life [it] would not have so much both pathos and the cosmic joke part. I made it up . . . 4000 years ago this happened. Here is this native going through this tropical forest. He had been doing this for a long time and he is singing as he goes. Well, a banana from a bunch fell down as he was walking and he slipped on it and broke his hip. Of course, the conclusion is "bananas break hips." There is the evidence. So naturally nobody wants their hips broken so the caring people started campaigning against bananas. Well, they managed to succeed because they did all kinds of research about how horrible bananas were for you and so on. Anyway, they finally got the whole population to buy the fact that bananas break hips, so bananas were banished.

3999 years later, when . . . they were teaching it in the seminars and all that–a little boy came from someplace. Nobody saw him come, did not know from where he came. He picks a banana and starts to eat it. The horrified population looks: "When is his hip going to break?" Because it would have to. And it did not. They said, "It will break in the next ten minutes. But in ten minutes it did not break. And . . . about a month went by and not only did he not have a broken hip, but he began to look so healthy. Now the wise ones among that group said, "You know, maybe we made a mistake"–3999 years later–Maybe bananas do not break hips." Well, gradually, that began to permeate and that is why we can eat bananas today.

Now . . . just change the content–put sex in it, for an example, put in mistakes. We have a whole lore about this, and this is what we try to do. So weave [the lessons of this story] into your wise, creative things.

Reframing Self Doubts

Now when we are asked to believe that A causes B, we are asked to be stupid. We are asked to turn our back on our experience. We are constantly told when we are kids, "Oh yes, you are just too little, [or] well that really doesn't work." Now once in a while you will do something so great it will bowl everybody over and they will say, "Well, you know, you really do have an idea." But it is not only with children because [after we grow up] we retain this idea that maybe what we are going to do is stupid. Tell me, how many have done that? [Arms raise]. All right. Just remember now, do not give yourself a black mark. First give yourself a gold star for being a good student, and then another gold star for finding out that you went to a college that did not prepare you too well, and another gold star for looking for what you can use instead.

Double-Level Messages to Ourselves

So, here we are then. We have to believe–give lip service to–something we believe does not fit our experience. Now what does that do? That tells us to be crazy. We have to say to ourselves that what we believe is not there, what we saw is not there. So when father comes home stumbling drunk and I say [something], mother says, "No, no, do not talk like that about him. He is just sick." Well, we know where that [kind of instruction from mother would] come from but as children we do not know that. [Or,] mother is raging and ranting and the father says, "She loves you." What do we do? We have to prostitute our experience, turn schizophrenic on one level because we cannot count on our experience. We can not even see the flaws of our own experience because if it does not fit somebody else's it is already wrong to begin with.

So, what price do we pay for that? Having to stuff down our unique- ness, our originality, our discovery; to deny our own experience which is the worst possible thing that can happen. And yet, all of this is done in love with the hope that we will be good people. [As a result] we have to behave double level. Now the smart ones among us say, "Ok, over there I will tell that story, over here I will tell that story. And when therapists find that out they call it "manipulation," while I call it survival.

That is why I bring everybody [in a family] together: so we can cut out the games–[the games of] forcing ourselves to say black is white and [trying to say it in a] believable way.

Remember to Think About Your Conclusions

I would like to suggest that many of the conclusions that we have arrived at through our so-called academic and professional theoretical base [from which] human beings [draw] are made up [like those of] that native in the forest. What I would like you to do is to look at the conclu- sions you have made–put them together. Do they really fit experience? That is why I keep saying taste everything, but swallow only that which fits. Ask yourself [about] every conclusion you have that goes like this, "That is the way it is."

When you hear yourself say, "That is the way it is," perk up your ears. Because the chances are pretty good that is how "it" *was* a hundred years ago and it has no effect now. But look at it. Look at all the stuff we are doing all the time, all the so-called psychological stuff. Some of it is absolutely fine, and when I put it to a test I can use it. Do that for yourself.

Attitude Toward Change

"Resistance"–Security and Keeping the Status Quo

. . . now when we get to here, the attitude towards change, [the auto- matic reflex] is to keep the status quo. Now, why? Because anything in the future is fearsome. You do not know what you are going to get into. You might fail. And you do not want to have a mistake. And, besides, the pain of the present is much more familiar than the possibility of the pain of the future . . . Keep the status quo.

Now this becomes a survival issue. Keep it as it is. Anybody who is trying to help people encounters something they call "resistance." I want to give you a new way to look at resistance. I want you to bless it every time you see it. Resistance is what I call you not knowing what I want you to do. That is the first one. You are not doing what I want you to do, that is your resistance. For you, resistance is having something really ok before you leave what you have got. It is the way you bless yourself to keep your survival. I never break down resistance, that is why I pay no attention to it. I go over here and I start putting in the other things. And then someone says, "You know, they are not really resistant." I say, "Why should they be?" "Aren't there some of you who were taught that you ought to have resistance"? Resistance will be in terms of how you see it, and I see it as a blessing. In fact, I feel if people are not offering me any resistance I wonder what is happening.

So that gets reframed, "resistance," to try to keep what I believe in where I feel safe. That is the story of the old prisoner that came out of prison after 20 years who slept on a bed of nails every night. When he got out of prison, he couldn't stand it to sleep on a bed because it was so familiar to have the bed of nails. Familiarity is far more potent than comfort. We are not oriented to comfort, we are oriented to familiarity. And it takes a whole new set of learnings to be oriented to comfort and happiness. We all want it, but it is a whole new set.

So what do we have, then? We have all the efforts to maintain a status quo. Security [pointing toward linear model on blackboard] is keeping things exactly as they are, is keeping the status quo. The energy is going into that. What happens is that all the energy has to be confined and formed and reformed within the same area.

REFERENCES

Banmen, J. and Satir, V. (1983) *Virginia Satir verbatim.* John Banmen Delta Psychological Associates, Inc. 11213 Canyon Crescent, North Delta, British Columbia, Canada V4E 2R6.

Brothers, B.J. (1996). From Virginia Satir: Ways of viewing the world; Explanation of events and attitude toward change. *Journal of Couples Therapy, 6* (1/2).

Brothers, B.J. (1996). Styles of Thinking: Comment on Virginia Satir's "Ways of viewing the world." *Journal of Couples Therapy, 6* (1/2).

Satir, V. et al. (1991). *The Satir model.* Palo Alto, California: Science and Behavior Books.

Satir, V. (1994). From Virginia Satir: Beyond the threat/reward model. In B. J. Brothers (Ed.), *Surpassing threats and rewards* (pp 1-7). Binghamton, New York: The Haworth Press, Inc.

Satir, V. (1995). Ways of viewing the world: Beyond the dominance and submission model. In B. J. Brothers (Ed), *Power and Partnering* (pp.1-14). Binghamton, New York: The Haworth Press, Inc.

Resistance in Couple Therapy: An Integration of Analytic and Systemic Approaches

Martin Astor
Robert Sherman

SUMMARY. The therapist in couple therapy needs to deal with resistances emerging from individual needs for defensive behavior as well as the systemic patterns such as co-dependency or the need to balance the system. Some types and sources of resistance stemming from individual fears and personality are defined. Some sources of resistance due to issues in intimacy are briefly described. Therapists need to analyze individual resistances and transferences. Techniques for dealing with resistance and positive ways for utilizing its energy are briefly presented within such categories as joining, deflecting, emphasizing the positive, educating, and bringing the reluctant client into therapy. An illustrative case study is provided. *[Article copies available for a fee from The Haworth Document Delivery Service: 1-800-342-9678. E-mail address: getinfo@haworth.com]*

INTRODUCTION

There is a way to buy a house and a way not to buy a house. If you "really" want the house, you are likely to buy it no matter what the price

Martin Astor, EdD, is Associate Emeritus Professor at Queens College, City University of New York, where for many years he was head of the Mental Health Counseling Program. He is currently a Director of the New York Society for Bioenergetic Analysis and he has a private clinical practice in New York City.

Robert Sherman, EdD, is Professor Emeritus at Queens College, Flushing, NY. He is in private practice as a consultant and supervisor.

[Haworth co-indexing entry note]: "Resistance in Couple Therapy: An Integration of Analytic and Systemic Approaches." Astor, Martin, and Robert Sherman. Co-published simultaneously in *Journal of Couples Therapy* (The Haworth Press, Inc.) Vol. 7, No. 1, 1997, pp. 9-25; and: *When One Partner Is Willing and the Other Is Not* (ed: Barbara Jo Brothers) The Haworth Press, Inc., 1997, pp. 9-25. Single or multiple copies of this article are available for a fee from The Haworth Document Delivery Service [1-800-342-9678, 9:00 a.m. - 5:00 p.m. (EST). E-mail address: getinfo@haworth.com].

or condition. Whereas if you are "really" not ready to buy, you are likely to find many good reasons for passing it by. This is the "really ready" principle: If you are "really ready" to make something work, it often works; and if you are not "really ready" to make it work, it often won't. This kind of decision-making may be conscious or unconscious. It's not usually easy for individuals to make momentous commitments, and it's even more complicated when couples try to do so. *Resistance to commitment*–to making a big move, changing, living with someone, getting married or divorced, or having children–is a critical factor in couple therapy.

In this article we seek to deal with the issues of resistance in couple therapy by integrating both psychodynamic and systemic theories, reflecting our belief that therapy must deal with both individual and couple dynamics. First, we will briefly describe the rationale for integrating psychodynamic and systemic models. Second, we will discuss the nature of resistance, psychodynamically and systemically. Third, we will look briefly at issues of intimacy that trigger resistance. Fourth, we will present a number of techniques and tactics that can be used to deal with it. And finally we will present an illustrative case.

RATIONALE FOR INTEGRATION

When couples first come to therapy, each party typically arrives having fully rehearsed a litany of complaints about what's wrong with the other. They point fingers and say things like, "He isn't interested in sex," "She doesn't understand me," "He's always working on some pet project and is never available," "She doesn't know how to handle the children." Soon it becomes evident that blame is a means of distancing themselves from each other. At the early stages, neither partner is "really ready" to make it work. It even seems as if each partner in the dyad is fighting against any possibility of intimacy or commitment. They each want the therapist "to fire" the other. Instead of recognizing that their respective personal issues are triggered when they enter a relationship, they find it easier to blame each other, and to focus on the other person's faults. They resist looking at themselves and their own emotional struggles. They unconsciously resist healing the presenting problem–the dysfunctional dyad.

Each partner comes to the relationship with individual motivations, expectations, beliefs, defenses, personality, and character. These include myths and unconscious attitudes about what marriage should be and expectations of entitlements that go with being a spouse. The couple then creates a pattern of interaction and communication driven by these factors, including roles and rules–and also including the maladaptive behavior that finally lands them in the therapist's office. This is the couple system.

Allen (1988), Sherman and Dinkmeyer (1987), and Wachtel and Wachtel (1986) are among those who have described the importance of working with both individual and the systemic patterns of interaction. There are three major categories of influences that evolve to shape a couple's behavior and their resistances in therapy: the meanings ascribed to past events, the current situation as each perceives it, and anticipation of the future. However, people do not live in their heads alone.

We are members of many conflicting subcultures and systems, each with its own identity, expectations, values, rules and regulations governing who we are *supposed* to be and how we are *supposed* to behave. Among them are age, gender, race, ethnicity, religion, peer groups, occupation, and the enterprise in which we work (Sherman, Shumsky, and Rountree, 1994).

Gergen (1991) and Lifton (1994) address this problem and claim that maintaining a single integrative self may be impossible or dysfunctional in our current social milieu. The person needs to be creative enough to develop constantly evolving multiple selves in each situation and system. It is obviously difficult to dance among the differences. We believe that the healthy person is one who can keep in mind who he is in all of these situations and how he will choose to participate in them. These subcultures and systems are not machines. They are created by people dynamically each moment. We therefore have a two way channel in which systems make strong demands upon and influence the personality and behavior of individuals and individuals act to shape the functioning of systems.

Therapists who work in couples counseling are also working with individuals. The skilled couples therapist is flexible and needs to understand what is going on in the couple system as well as in each of the individuals within that system. In all kinds of group work we have to know what each of the individuals involved are thinking and feeling, and how they are separately affected by the group process. Couple therapy is always more effective when we work in both directions simultaneously–from the couple to the individual and back again to the couple. Often the therapist may need to see the individual in a private session, or the therapist may focus on an individual during the couple session. This combined dynamic of working interchangeable with couple and individual and in an integrated approach combining analytic and systemic theory will inevitably yield optimal therapeutic results.

INDIVIDUAL DYNAMICS IN COUPLE RESISTANCE

In an earlier paper, "Therapeutic neurosis: the need to resist the healing process in psychotherapy," Astor argued that resistance in therapy is actually necessary (Astor, 1994). Resistance is always to be expected in any kind of therapy, and in fact "optimal resistance" is healthy and positive whenever it becomes necessary for the client to defend or protect him or her self. Resistance most often occurs when change is about to take place, tending to surface whenever the client is trying to stop the process of self exploration, examination, or illumination. Early, historic defense mechanisms quickly come into play in the service of resistance.

FORMS OF RESISTANCE

Resistance in therapy may take many forms: antagonism, lateness, fear, non-cooperation, self-hatred, refusal to take responsibility, and so on. Although difficult to work with, oppositional behavior and negativity often hold great potential for growth and change. Conscious resistance may occur because of shame and fear, whereas unconscious resistance may manifest as refusal to yield for fear of pain, abandonment, loss of love and loss of control. Defenses like (Freud, 1946) projection, rationalization, denial, and displacement are still needed to support the ego when it feels threatened or overwhelmed. Defenses work in flux with resistance to protect the ego from awareness of unacceptable ideation and conflicts.

Anderson and Stewart (1983) described many forms of resistance including resistance to entering therapy, contract-related resistance, challenges to the therapist's competence, and resistance created by helping therapists and institutions. We cannot discuss all the many ways in which resistance occurs in this brief article.

In couple therapy, resistance may be unconscious and irrational and even serve to perpetuate neurotic defenses. This may result in repression of memories, feelings, and fantasies that the client finds too powerful to accept as part of him or her self. This can further result in negative transference toward his or her spouse and the therapist, causing the client to defeat, spite and sabotage the therapeutic process.

In studying the nature of resistance it is important to differentiate between the concepts of personality and character. Personality refers to an individual's predictable, persistent patterns of behavior. Most of us have regular, daily and weekly routines, and most of our behaviors become repetitive and predictable over time. More pointedly, personality–persona– is a mask. It's the way we consistently show ourselves to the world. Character, on the other hand, is what we really are in our bones. An outgrowth of our "becoming," it reflects our deepest values. It is also, of course, the result of our individual histories of nurture and nature. Resistance is more a function of personality; whereas defenses generally stem from our characterological nature. We can change personality more easily than character. At the outset of therapy working through resistance helps clients to try new masks and to overcome negativity, cynicism, and hopelessness. For more permanent change to occur, however, we need to work in depth with the mechanisms of defense. The latter is a much slower process.

We can also look at resistance and defense from an energetic point of view (Freud, 1946). In physics, resistance is what converts energy to heat. Resistance is inversely related to conductance–it is impedance, retardant of change and movement, serving to maintain the status quo. Analogously, defenses use psychic energy when they operate in the service of resistance.

Modes of defense arise from character instinctively, for they are related to early developmental life experiences as well as to genetic factors. As clients change character to function better in their relationships, they become less defensive, more trusting and respectful. As they achieve better characterological health and greater understanding of themselves, they become better able to commit to their relationships and to tolerate the necessary give and take. Rogers (1961) points out that, as people feel less threatened they eventually feel sufficiently secure to drop their defenses, to become more open and better able to look into themselves. As they learn to accept and respect themselves, having dropped their defenses, they become less resistant to life and to relationships with significant others. The energy formerly tied up in defenses and resistances can then be reclaimed, affording greater pleasure in life and greater capacity to give pleasure to others. They learn what is axiomatic in couple therapy, that the best way to change the other is to change one's own behavior. Of course, the other then has to cooperate by also changing his or her behavior.

COUPLES DYNAMICS IN TREATING RESISTANCE: ISSUES OF INTIMACY

Issues of intimacy arise due to differences in beliefs, expectations, myths, styles, individual needs, poor communication, and to conflicts over roles or distribution of power in the relationship. Simplistically stated, "If you don't behave as I expect, you couldn't really love me, especially since I am right and you are wrong. Therefore, I have to protect myself from hurt and harm." Thus a negative pattern of interactive behaviors evolves and is reinforced as each partner repeatedly assumes his or her defensive position.

The couple does not necessarily have to be in conflict for resistance to arise. One partner may be suffering from a mental or physical disorder, addiction, or life-adjustment problem. Resistance reflects the ways the other partner may be reinforcing the symptomatic behavior, or how the symptomatic behavior helps to maintain the dyadic system. For example, we may have a violent husband and a depressed wife. The presenting symptom is the wife's depression. We may discover that, when the wife is depressed, the husband is less violent and more nurturing. She will soon resist giving up her depression because of fear of her husband's violence, which she may not even mention in the therapy. Following are ten categories of intimacy issues common in couples.

Territoriality: Beliefs and feelings about emotional and physical space are at odds. What one partner considers comfortable is utterly suffocating or too distant for the other. Resistance serves to protect one person's space and boundaries or lessens the need to fight to reduce the other's.

Intensity: One partner is very passionate and emotive and regards the other as cold, withdrawn, not in touch with feelings. The second partner thinks the first is too intense, hysterical, or crazy.

Styles: Some like it hot, some like it cool. Some like it bright, others dimmer. Some prefer more social companionship, others less. There are preferred and habitual styles of speech and dress, ways of thinking, expressions of humor, and many more. Identity is bound up with these styles and must be protected.

Gender Differences: Men and women are reared somewhat differently and have different approaches to intimacy. Thus, in couples women tend to prefer *being* together and engaging in lots of cooperative personal talk. Men tend to prefer *doing* things together, focusing on achievement and competition; and for intimacy they enjoy more physical presence as well as sexual intercourse. Women fear being omitted, discounted, unjoined, or overpowered in the relationship. Men fear they will be unappreciated, demeaned, or made to feel failure, with loss of face or power.

Symbiotic Attunement: This is the elusive art of knowing exactly what the other is thinking or feeling. The demand that "You must know me without my telling you what I need, think, or feel" leads to a great deal of disappointment and conflict. The disappointment is experienced by one, usually the woman, almost as if the self is being obliterated. The other, usually the man, feels assaulted and a failure. Defenses are mounted by both.

Differences in Rules, Customs, and Traditions: Both partners try to establish rules about how they are to function based on their assumptive values and backgrounds. Are they allowed to vent anger or must they swallow it to keep the peace at any price? Are holidays to be celebrated with extended family or by going on vacation or out to dinner? Failure to accept and behave *my way* is rejection of *me.*

Demands That the Other Make Major Changes in Personality and Behavior: Demands that a partner change cause that partner to feel disrespected and rejected, eliciting defensive, negative responses and a strong resistance to change–after all, it seems like giving up personhood. Meanwhile, the one who makes demands probably feels discounted, unloved and frustrated.

Being of Several Minds: Some people bounce back and forth between the fear of being abandoned and the fear of being absorbed. They alternately reach out for and reject closeness. Those who were physically or emotionally abused or neglected by people close to them may strongly desire intimacy yet be terrified that the closest person is the very one who will somehow betray and abuse them. Defenses are erected as protection against such fears, usually by alternately inviting and then pushing the partner away.

Reciprocally, Negative Role Relationships: Individuals assume roles in their relationships, and sometimes in life in general. Some examples (among hundreds) are: the aggressor, controller, pleaser, helpless one, rebellious child, tragedy king or queen, inspector general, or ill one. Each person behaves in a way so as to maintain the other's behavior reciprocally, e.g., the rescuer and the needy one. Neither role can truly exist without the other; they are complementary. The resistance arises because each believes that if he or she does any less or differently, the situation will be measurably worse.

Sexuality: Sexual behavior and personal identity have been so closely intertwined in our culture that many fears about self-adequacy are related to sex. For that reason, sex makes an excellent weapon for one partner to use against the other, through overt physical aggression, emotional demeaning, or withholding of sexual participation. Some believe that sex is dirty or immoral, and that engaging in it even when married is wrong. A few of the many other sources of distress eliciting defensive behavior are: differences in preferences about what may or may not be done, or the sequence; morning vs. night person; fear of being seen, heard, or known to be engaging in sex; fear of pregnancy; fear of diseases; fear of loss of control, power, or even of self. For a more detailed description of issues in intimacy see Sherman, Oresky, and Rountree (1991). This book also contains a chapter on resistance.

All of the above categories can constitute very powerful internal and interactive forces that may seem tantamount to psychological life or death, and therefore can evoke very great resistance to change. Still, because of their very strength, it is often possible to lay bare those forces, to examine the resistance, then convert its abundant energy to constructive use. Secondary gain–the benefits that occur from a neurosis–may serve to further strengthen resistance. Only successful negotiation of all those dynamics central to the problem will enable the "working-through" process to occur. The working-through process requires helping the client replace blind repetition of neurotic, dysfunctional behavior with more developmentally mature and appropriate behavior.

Couple therapy, to be successful, requires careful analysis of multiple transferences and countertransference (Freud, 1924). Each partner in the relationship needs to better understand how his or her own resistance works and inhibits change. As clients come to understand the meaning of their respective resistances, they gradually develop the strength to go through the pain of changing. Instead of finger-pointing and blaming the other member of the dyad for whatever isn't working, they become better able to look into themselves and their motives. Through proper analysis of resistance, understanding its meaning and how it works, the partners eventually learn to take appropriate responsibility for developing and maintaining a healthy and meaningful relationship.

In addition to analyzing resistance and transference, there are many techniques and tactics available for working with resistance. Following are some general ones that can be readily adapted to specific purposes. The reader is cautioned that it is not our intention to provide a bag of tricks. Rather we are briefly summarizing techniques that have been successfully used and reported in the literature and that we know, from our own extensive clinical experience (at least 75 years combined), to be particularly effective in working with resistance. The reader is urged to use professional judgment based on theory as well as the specifics of the situation in applying any of the following techniques and tactics.

TECHNIQUES AND TACTICS

We can move in many directions to work with resistance and build upon its own power and energy. We can join clients to reframe meanings, interpret beliefs and behavior, give feedback on consequences of beliefs and behavior. We can describe, externalize, normalize, imitate, and dramatize implications and complications resulting from their belief systems. We can devise paradoxical statements or prescriptions and educate clients in conflict-resolution skills. We can use bibliotherapy to evoke new sympathy and understanding of self and other, and make up fairy tales, do symbolic exorcisms, and record audio-videotape sessions for playback of useful parts. We can employ imagery-visualizations to help work through fears and foster greater self-love. We can work with role reversals and story completions. We can make use of "objective" tests and inventories and do tracking, focusing on the positives, focusing on what has been successful in the past, and encourage appropriate self-disclosure. We will group many of these techniques and tactics into five categories and briefly elaborate on them.

Joining

Often a client resists therapy because he or she does not agree with the direction it is taking, or with an assignment made, or feels that an undesired agreement has been forced. Other times there are competing values. For example, the wife may be working with the therapist in a direction desirable to her, while the husband's competing value draws him in another direction. This causes one or both to sabotage the work or to alternately go forward and backward. Further, the therapist may be pursuing a goal different from both clients, or may have accepted a goal of one partner that is adverse to the goal of the other. Following are five ways to join with the couple.

The therapist can reassess the goals of the therapy with the clients and seek new cooperative agreements about what they want to accomplish together. What is each willing to do to achieve a common goal defined in positive terms? For example, "what can we each do to have more pleasant time together when we are both so pressed for time?"

The therapist can acknowledge and validate the clients' positions by saying, "I can understand why you would think, feel, or do that, coming from where you are." Of course, acknowledgement by the therapist does not necessarily mean agreement.

We can track behavior carefully to find out where it is coming from and what it means and to explore its consequences. For example, "If this is so, then what, then what . . .," until it is clear.

We can "translate" constructively the feelings and demands of each partner for the other. The therapist might interpret: "What Jane is saying is that she cares for you very much, but because of what happened she is having difficulty trusting what you say, and she needs help with that."

Reframing is another way of recasting negative beliefs into a more positive framework. In working with a woman who complains that her husband is boring, the therapist might reflect: "So, your husband is a very stable person who likes to spend his leisure time at home rather than run around a lot."

Emphasizing the Positive

The clients are typically "You"-ing and faulting each other in their conflict.

The therapist can soften the climate by asking them to recall their first meeting and what impressed each about the other; and what was attractive and impressive in subsequent meetings and in the decision to come together as a couple. This is also a good way to elicit the hidden contract between them and how it is currently being challenged.

The therapist can also ask such questions as: "What do you currently respect and admire about your partner? What positive things does your partner contribute to this family? To others? What are all the interests and values that you share together? Could you please list the decisions you made together this week? Is it possible that the differences between you constitute only a small fraction of all that goes on between you? What have you done in the past to solve these problems, or make them less severe, that has worked? Was there a time when you could either avoid or solve these conflicts, or when they didn't exist?" These questions help put the negatives and the relationship itself in a more positive perspective, and can demonstrate that the partners have had many experiences of getting along and even in solving problems.

Deflecting the Resistance

When the therapy sessions with the couple appear to be very toxic, to worsen rather than ameliorate the conflict, there are many options the therapist can choose for deflecting the resistance and moving the work forward.

Perhaps the most powerful is to work with the families of origin as described by Kerr and Bowen (1988), Framo (1992), and Freeman (1992). The theory is that the old business of growing up and family legacies and loyalties are at the root of the present dysfunction, and are involved in the contagion of anxiety, fusions and lack of differentiation. Each multigenerational family of origin is thus examined in great detail and, if possible, brought in for collaborative sessions to work out the unresolved issues. (For purposes of reducing resistance, the number of sessions required may be far fewer than anticipated by the above writers.)

Setting up analogous experiences is another way to detoxify immediate interactions. Reading poems, stories, or novels; listening to specific songs; or seeing a particular play or movie may help the couple to get a different perspective on their own situation and behavior.

Having the partners write to each other, rather than fighting it out or holding it in, often affords them a more reasoned form of communication that is less reactive or not on "automatic" responses. We are usually more careful and considered about what we write than about what we say.

Taking time to write it also breaks the pattern of spontaneous, impulsive responses.

The family sculpting technique enables the therapist and the couple to visually perceive what is going on in the couple's relationship by interpreting their behaviors in physical interaction (Sherman and Fredman, 1986). Each partner may be asked to set up the sculpture as he or she is experiencing it. The therapist asks "What would be a better arrangement for each of you? Work it out non-verbally." There are many variations.

It may be useful to prescribe the Couple Conference (Manaster and Corsini, 1982), in which the couple devotes a ritual time and place to talking to each other, one at a time without interruptions; to revealing the self to the other without trying to solve anything. Usually each speaks 30 minutes uninterrupted, followed by the partner speaking similarly at least once a week, set up as a ritual.

The "empty chair" can help a client talk to him or her self, or talk to the other indirectly, either to practice more constructive or effective communication or better to understand buried feelings and beliefs.

Role reversal can be employed to help sensitize the partners to each other. The therapist coaches them until each one really starts "being" the other and feeling what that is like. The therapist asks: "Be your partner now and respond in his or her shoes to what you just did or said. Get into what it really feels like by your partner to experience that."

Objective tests and inventories can serve as external "authority" to help clients better know themselves and each other. These take matters out of the realm of morality and defense to that of "objective" information (Fredman and Sherman, 1987).

Moving from Emotion to Reason and New Skills Through Education

Couples may be stuck in a resistant pattern because they don't know any other way to cope. People can only choose among known options and available skills and bodies of knowledge.

The therapist can teach clients conflict-resolution skills such as the Negotiating Guide (Sherman, Oresky, and Rountree, 1991). Clients are encouraged to view differences between them as normal and expected, and to understand that it is legitimate to disagree. Understanding that, they have come to respectfully find a way to resolve their legitimate differences through giving in to each other graciously; making a deal or compromise arrived at through proposals and counter-proposals rather than demands; taking their conflict to a higher level of needs and goals–e.g., We both really want to find some way of having more time together, rather than, Why can't we go out to dinner on Sundays?; and, failing all else, letting fate decide—by the highest card, choosing odds or evens, picking a straw, flipping a coin—with the loser giving in graciously.

As an adjunct to therapy, clients can be referred to couple-enrichment groups, A.A., or other program groups, parent-education groups, and other classes or readings, to help them learn better communication or other specific skills.

To keep matters clear and fresh in their minds, clients can be requested to write brief notes at the conclusion of each session in an ongoing therapy journal, recording particular things that impressed them, home tasks agreed on, or other agreements made. Or the couple can be requested to write up a contract embodying whatever agreements have been made. The contract should be posted in a very prominent place at home. Also, at the end of the session the clients may be asked to summarize orally what they got out of it. At the beginning of the following session they can similarly be asked what impressed them in the past meeting and what they did with it.

Getting the Reluctant Client into Therapy

There are many techniques a therapist uses to involve a partner who refuses to come in for therapy. A few follow.

One partner shows up alone and claims that the other refuses to come. We have found that sometimes this is resistance on the part of the one who comes, who really doesn't want the other partner there. In addition to exploring this possibility, permission is requested to telephone the missing partner. Very often, a simple invitation from the therapist is sufficient to bring the person in.

It is possible to include the absent member by sharing the session with him or her. This can be done by asking the one present to describe the session in detail to the other either orally or by writing an account of it. Similarly, the therapist can write to the absent member and request permission to send a written summary of each session in order to keep him or her informed assuming that he or she is vitally interested in the process. Following a number of such communications, the person may again be invited to join the sessions.

Call the absent member and simply begin a conversation. Ask a few non-threatening questions about the partner, then ask about reactions to the partner. Finally, ask whether the person is willing to join the sessions, or at least respond to occasional phone calls.

When the resistant one pleads too little time, he or she can be invited to join in via speaker phone in the therapist's office. Some therapists in New York currently use a van to pick up busy people at their offices, then conduct the sessions in the van. Home visits are also a possibility.

Finally, the therapist can telephone the absent partner and inform him or her that "Your partner is talking about you and representing you in particular ways. Wouldn't you like to come in and present your side of the story so that I can get a more objective picture?"

CASE EXAMPLE OF COUPLE RESISTANCE

Let us examine a case to explore how resistance between two individuals has arisen. We will look at the dynamics involved in working with resistance and make suggestions for effective treatment.

Woman: I was married twice before, and now–the third time around–I really want to make this marriage work. But my husband seems to be obsessed with his work and he's not romantic. I've had lovers on and off since we were married, because my husband seems to have a very low sex drive. He doesn't know about my trysts, and he could never accept them. I do it on the sly. I love my husband and I really want to work it out with him, yet I'm not willing to give up my love affairs.

Man: I love my wife very much, but she's always complaining and always running off to shop or to be with her friends. I try to get her involved with my work. I'm rebuilding an old house, but she never wants to come with me to help. I like being with her, but she's always running away from the house so much. I can't understand why she complains about me. I give her everything she wants and I love her company.

Analysis

The woman in this case is not "really ready" to work through a meaningful relationship with her husband if she still resists giving up her lover. She has ambivalence toward her husband; she's angry at him, frustrated by his preoccupation with working on their house. And yet she needs him for security and dependability since she fears a third divorce and being alone in the world without support. She knows that her marriage isn't working, but she isn't allowing it to work so long as she keeps her lover. She cannot fully accept her husband, nor can she take in his love, no matter what he does to accommodate her. On some level the husband feels rejected by the wife, and he behaves accordingly. The more he seems to ignore her, the more she is dissatisfied. As her frustration increases, she turns to other men. Thus, her feeling that she has a dysfunctional marriage is confirmed. Neither husband nor wife is moving or changing; nor is either able to receive any satisfaction from the marital relationship.

The husband is operating in the dark. He doesn't know about his wife's lover. He feels something is wrong, but he can't put his finger on it. Although the therapist knows about it, the husband can't be told since the wife asked for confidentiality. The therapist is in a dilemma about keeping this important information a secret.

The therapist decides to confront the wife about her resistance to giving up her lover. He tells her that no authentic marriage counseling or therapy can be accomplished while she's still acting out sexually with another man. He can see her for individual therapy, but he can't work in couples therapy and still protect her "secret." In other words, the therapist advises her to make a commitment to get "really ready" to work on her marriage.

During individual sessions with the wife it is learned that she's had a long history of physical health issues. She suffered various cancers and blood conditions, for which she's been frequently hospitalized, and her mother died of cancer at an early age. The client was raised by her father, who was a gambler and an alcoholic. As a result of discussing these many issues, the client soon comes to realize why security with a man is such an important issue in her life. As for this third marriage, she's settled on a man who offers very little romance, but much security. He is a stable, hard working person. In her individual therapy she also learns that the kind of romantic relationships she enjoys in her trysts is developmentally imma-ture. She acts out with these men as if she is a teenager, and in fact, she soon comes to realize that she really is trying to relive her lost teen years. Because her mother died early, the client had been responsible for the care of her younger brother and her irresponsible father. In effect she never had a chance to enjoy her teen years. Armed with these insights, she eventually is able to make a full commitment to her husband, and to give up her lover(s). In time she renegotiates her relationship with her husband, and thereby rebuilds her marriage.

A few individual sessions with the husband revealed that he is a recent immigrant and that he comes from a large eastern European family. Al-though he was trained as an engineer, he is unable to get a professional license to work in the United States largely due to his very poor English. At first, he worked almost at a minimum-wage level. He has been married before, and divorced, and has joint custody of a ten-year-old son. While his family in Europe holds high expectations of him, he feels himself to be a failure.

Although his marriage is dysfunctional, he clings to his wife for many reasons. She is beautiful, she is an American, she has a good job, and she is creative, exotic and articulate. He literally worships her. In many ways she is his ticket to establishing economic viability in a new and strange environment. Thus she, in her own way, offers him a great deal of security. The fact of the matter is, husband and wife are co-dependents.

Having come to these realizations and insights in his individual sessions the man strives more and more to free himself from his dependency. He concentrates on improving his language skills, he studies for and passes the examination to become a licensed building contractor. He becomes more actively involved in his wife's life. In time he is able to make more demands on her. On some unconscious level his new behavior has the effect of dissuading her from carrying on relationships with other men.

Following individual work, subsequent sessions with the couple became extremely effective. Both parties are newly committed to the marriage. During the couple sessions, several major techniques were used to deal with the resistance endemic to their system. First, the couple was asked to sculpt what it was like to be in this relationship. Then they were asked to feel what it is like to be in the other's place as the other is experiencing the marriage. This gave them some insight into each others' feelings and experiences. Second, the husband was asked if he was tired of being the responsible one always working at home. Wouldn't he like to put some of his bountiful energy to work by being responsible for the fun and romance in the marriage while the wife took on more responsibilities for the home. She was asked if she wouldn't want to make her home a place she really wanted to enjoy. With some coaching they accepted and integrated this role reversal into their pattern of interaction. Third, the issue of the fear of intimacy was addressed by prescribing with their agreement to the couple conference. Giving them a structured ritual made it more safe to share themselves and learn to be emotionally intimate.

The systemic marital dynamics are changed. The two are no longer co-dependent and they have each gained in respect for the other. Both partners are aware of their own life-long issues and are better able to enter a committed relationship. Instead of blaming one another for things that go awry, they have learned to take responsibility for their own behaviors. They still have issues, they still have problems, but they know what they need to do to make their system work.

CONCLUSION

This article has taken a position between two theoretical extremes–that there is no such thing as resistance, and that everything in therapy revolves around resistance. We believe that some resistance is a normal occurrence in individual and couple therapy. We further believe that resistance is a protective strategy of individual character, personality and motivation that is elicited and reinforced in systemic patterns of interaction. Individuals together create systems and systems strongly influence their individual members. Therefore we have endeavored to present an integrative approach to dealing with resistance involving both individual and couple systems.

We asserted that, to deal with resistance the therapist must analyze it with each member as well as analyze both the transference and counter-transference in the therapeutic system. We described five categories of techniques and tactics that therapists can employ to harness the positive energy of resistance for positive growth and change: (1) Joining; (2) Emphasizing the positive; (3) Deflecting the resistance; (4) Moving from emotion to reason and developing new skills through education; (5) Getting the reluctant client into therapy; and finally, we presented a case to illustrate how we have treated resistance in couples therapy using an integrative approach that addresses both psyche and system.

AUTHOR NOTE

Martin Astor has published numerous articles in psychotherapy, bioenergetic analysis, hypnoanalysis and transpersonal counseling. He is planning a paper on the psychology of pottery–or getting hooked on clay. Address: 301 East 69th Street, Apt. 5L, New York, NY 10021-5513.

Robert Sherman is author of many articles and five books on family therapy. His most recent book is *Enlarging the therapeutic circle: The therapist's guide to collaborative therapy with families and schools* published by Brunner Mazel, 1994, with Adaia Shumsky and Yvonne Rountree. Address: 154-23A Riverside Drive, Beechhurst, NY 11357.

REFERENCES

Allen, D.M. (1988). *Unifying individual and family therapies.* San Francisco. Jossey-Bass.

Anderson, C. and Stewart S. (1983). *Mastering resistance. A practical guide to family therapy.* New York. Guilford Press.

Astor, M. (1992). Invisibility and character. *The Journal.* International Institute For Bioenergetic Analysis, 5, 1, 45-54.

Astor, M. (1994). Therapeutic neurosis: The need to resist the healing process in psychotherapy. *Journal of Contemporary Psychotherapy,* 24, 1, 39-50.

Framo, J. (1992). *Family-of-origin therapy: An intergenerational approach.* New York. Brunner Mazel.

Freeman, D.S. (1992). *Family therapy with couples. The family of origin approach.* Northvale, N.J. Jason Aronson.

Freud, A. (1946). *The ego and the mechanisms of defense.* New York: International Universities Press.

Freud, S. (1924). *The dynamics of transference.* (Vol II of Collected Papers). London: Hogarth Press, Institute of Psychoanalysis.

Gergen, K. (1991). *The saturated self. Delemmas of identity in contemporary life.* New York. Basic Books.

Kerr, M.E. and Bowen, M. (1988) Family evaluation: An approach based on Bowen's theory. New York: Norton.

Lifton, R.J. (1993) *The protean self. Human resilience in an age of fragmentation.* New York. Basic Books.

Lowen, A. (1982). *The will to live and the wish to die.* The International Institute of Bioenergetic Analysis, New York.

Manaster, G. and Corsini, R.C. (1982) Individual Psychology. *Theory and practice.* ITASCA, Il. Peacock.

Rogers, C. (1961). *On becoming a person.* Houghton Mifflin.

Sherman, R. (1993). Issues in intimacy and techniques for change: An Adlerian perspective. *Individual Psychology.* 49.3&4.318-329.

Sherman, R. and Dinkmeyer, D. (1987). *Systems of family therapy: An adlerian integration.* New York. Brunner Mazel.

Sherman, R., Oresky, P., and Rountree, Y. (1991). *Solving problems in couples and family therapy: techniques and tactics.* New York: Brunner Mazel.

Sherman, R., Shumsky, A. and Rountree, Y.B. (1994). *Enlarging the therapeutic circle. The therapist's guide to collaborative therapy with families and schools.* New York. Brunner Mazel.

Wachtel, P.L. and Wachtel, E. F. (1986). *Family Dynamics in individual therapy.* New York. Guilford.

The Power Struggle Stage:
From Polarization to Empathy

Liberty Kovacs

SUMMARY. The third stage of marriage presents the couple with one of the most difficult, and least understood, issues in the relationship–the issue of power. The author examines the dynamics of power and the therapeutic tools that have proven useful in defusing the intensity of the power struggles, thus freeing the couple to re-experience empathy and love for each other. *[Article copies available for a fee from The Haworth Document Delivery Service: 1-800-342-9678. E-mail address: getinfo@haworth.com]*

A couple trapped in a power struggle is recognizable from the moment they walk in the therapist's office. The coldness, the distance, and the pain are palpable. Neither is willing to speak first; each waits for the other. The silence is filled with resistance and tension. Finally, one shrugs and speaks the obvious: "We are not getting along. We fight all the time. We can't agree on anything."

Everything about the couple's behavior signals where they may be

Liberty Kovacs, PhD, MFCC, has been a marital therapist for over 25 years and is in private practice in Sacramento, CA. She has taught at the University of California, San Francisco and Davis, at the California State University, Sacramento, and she was a consultant with the Community Mental Health Program in Sacramento County. In addition to private practice, she is currently teaching workshops for couples based on her model (and videotape) of the six stages of marriage. This model was the subject of her PhD dissertation from the California Graduate School of Family Psychology.

[Haworth co-indexing entry note]: "The Power Struggle Stage: From Polarization to Empathy." Kovacs, Liberty. Co-published simultaneously in *Journal of Couples Therapy* (The Haworth Press, Inc.) Vol. 7, No. 1, 1997, pp. 27-37; and: *When One Partner Is Willing and the Other Is Not* (ed: Barbara Jo Brothers) The Haworth Press, Inc., 1997, pp. 27-37. Single or multiple copies of this article are available for a fee from The Haworth Document Delivery Service [1-800-342-9678, 9:00 a.m. - 5:00 p.m. (EST). E-mail address: getinfo@haworth.com].

developmentally in terms of their relationship: the tightness of their bodies, the cautious, measured speech, the avoidance of eye contact, the over-controlled emotions. With all these outward signs, the therapist may begin to hypothesize that a power struggle is one major issue. As soon as one starts to talk and the other sits in cold silence awaiting his/her turn, or one interrupts to disagree with the first statement, the therapist is almost certain the hypothesis is a valid one.

A few years ago, these two people fell in love and decided to spend the rest of their lives together. Now, they are on the brink of divorce. What happened to that love? What happened to the two people who could spend hours together talking and having fun? How did they arrive at this angry, hurt stalemate?

THEORETICAL FRAMEWORK

At this point let us review some of the main concepts in the model of marriage that I have called an integrated developmental and family systems model (Kovacs, 1988). Marriage is a dynamic and complex process that starts when two people "first lay eyes on each other" (Satir, 1964) and they decide to be together. This process continues to be dynamic and complex throughout the life of the marriage.

Marriage is complex because it is rooted in our unconscious needs, wants, expectations and conflict, which are, in turn, rooted in the early infant relationship with the mother and father, i.e., the way the child experienced the separation-individuation process, and the level of those achievements toward the development of a separate identity from that of the parents, sets the stage for future development and future relationships.

In the first separation-individuation process during the first three to five years, the psychic structures of the individual are laid out. This process of progressive differentiation and integration of the personality continues through adolescence when another major step toward differentiation occurs. The third evolutionary process of enormous proportions occurs in adulthood about every seven to ten years throughout the marital process. This process is continuous and contiguous with parenthood. One does not stop to wait for the other. Each transition or change that a couple experiences has the capacity to revive or recapitulate past conflicts or problems and provides an opportunity to rework and/or complete the "unfinished business" from the past.

Beside the separation-individuation process, the other building blocks of the marital relationship that contribute to its complexity are: the parents' models of marriage and the structure and process of each family of origin in which each individual grew up.

So, what does falling in love have to do with theories, concepts and therapeutic tools? Is falling in love Mother Nature's way of tricking us into getting married? Why do we marry our "worst nightmare" as August Napier (1978) suggested? Recent writers (Hendrix, 1988; Travers, 1991) emphasized that the unconscious purpose of marriage is to heal the wounds of childhood.

My observations of marital couples indicate that people fall in love with the person who will evoke the issues that were not completed in the early relationship with the parents. In order to complete the "unfinished business of the past," the factor that seems essential is that the person who is chosen as a mate/partner must exhibit on an unconscious level the traits of the parents that were perceived as negative and/or conflictual. Even the unresolved issues that the parents struggled with may get re-enacted in the battles of the married adult children.

On the other hand, needs for love and affection may lie dormant in the individuals until they meet the person who will awaken that dormant part of the personality. In the process of falling in love, the couple is building a reservoir (metaphorically speaking) in which to store their powerful emotions and passions and, thereafter, becomes a source of love and affection when the relationship runs dry or becomes distant and disengaged.

Overall, marriage is viewed as the next arena after adolescence in which the individuals develop a context in which their growth process is continued and where they achieve a consolidation of their identities as individuals. At the same time they are "growing a self," the couple is growing a couple identity as well.

THE EARLY STAGES OF MARRIAGE

During the Honeymoon stage, the emphasis of the two lovers was on maintaining their intense closeness and in nurturing their relationship. During the second stage, or Expectations, the couple is realizing how different they are in ways they communicate, think, feel and in their styles of working and completing tasks. They also are realizing that they need time apart to be with friends, family and co-workers. One or both feels the need for more independence and apartness from the partner, but s/he did not express these needs openly. Gradually, they have been moving out of a cocoon-like existence and expanding the boundaries of their relationship.

Now, in the third stage, the focus is shifting again; gently at first, then, picking up momentum. Each starts thinking, "Can I be myself in this relationship?" "Will s/he still love me if I express how I really feel? "What if I want to do something *my* way?" "What if I disagree?" "Will I be accepted?"

In order to answer these questions, each partner will have to assert him/herself, perhaps, in a way that has not been done before. One may feel anxious and fearful about trying something different. The other may have no qualms whatsoever about saying or doing what s/he wants, come what may.

In the early part of the third stage, one may tug in one direction and find that the other is pulling in a different direction. One may suggest a movie and they end up arguing about which movie to go to . . . or which restaurant to go for dinner. They may have their first argument over some "stupid little thing" and, then, wonder what all the fuss was about.

At first, their arguments appear "silly" and inconsequential on the surface, but something is brewing underneath. The relationship is becoming a testing ground for each spouse to assert him/herself in making decisions, in determining how the relationship will be structured and how tasks will be shared and completed. The struggles to resolve these issues are manifested in a range of interactions: from silence and withdrawal to tugs-of-war to polarization and all-out battles (from verbal to physical abuse). The marriage at this point appears to be heading for chaos and self-destruction. This is the time for testing the trust, love and acceptance that they have for each other and the relationship. They are shedding their facades and armor and allowing a little of the true self to peek through.

"Can I trust you to accept this part of my Self? As a child when I spoke up or wanted something my way, I got criticized (or punished or rejected)?" Everyone grows up in a family that is different and unique. How one asserts his/her individuality in the family varies with each family; how we express ourselves in a marriage will vary with each relationship. These issues of self-assertion and individuality in a relationship–"doing things my way"–propels the couple into the third stage of marriage which I have called the Power Struggle Stage.

The big complaints that therapists frequently hear during this stage are: "We can't communicate" and "We don't understand each other any longer." More demands are expressed which may escalate into angry accusations and blaming each other (for being "stubborn," "unreasonable," "emotional," or "illogical"). Confrontations become more frequent and polarization and chaos seem inevitable.

Each partner is now feeling confused, hurt, alone and scared. The issue is one of control and power and they don't know how to reach the other without "giving in" which is equated with "losing my Self again."

"To be or not to be (my Self)"–that is the question. "Do I give in or stand and fight?" "Will I lose again (like I did with father/mother)?" "How do I get accepted?" The dance the couple is performing is one of approach/withdraw. The pain is immense, but neither can bend or allow him/herself to feel vulnerable. The situation seems too threatening.

Yet for two people who love each other and who want to be together, the choice is paradoxical: in order to feel accepted, one must allow him/herself to be vulnerable to the other–to show the softer (or more independent) side of one's self. And that is so risky! "If this part of me was not accepted in my family, how can my partner accept me?"

Yes, that is the risk: to show another aspect of one's True Self, instead of attempting to control or overpower the other in order to get one's own way. The risk is to reveal one's vulnerable Self and, in turn, receive empathy, love and understanding.

To avoid this risk out of fear of rejection is to stay stuck in unending battles over who is right and who is wrong–over who will win and who will lose. These battles, at the very least, will distance the pair from each other and, at worst, will erode the relationship and destroy the trust and love. Couples who have been trapped in their power-struggle dances for years are sad, unhappy and very hurt people.

To resolve their power struggle, the couple must be willing to come together, to communicate their feelings, and negotiate their differences. Before describing the tasks that must be accomplished and the therapeutic tools that will be used to transform power struggles into empathetic, supportive interactions, the meaning of power in a relationship needs to be explored further.

MEANINGS OF POWER

What does power have to do with marriage? The answer is "Everything." Without power we cannot exist. Rollo May (1978) described power as a "fundamental aspect of the life process." When couples are asked what they associate with power, the usual responses are: "control," "authority," "strength," "influence," "dominance," "violence," and "aggression." Yes, these are one aspect of this complex issue which is manifested when one person, group or nation is trying to exert power and dominate another. Oftentimes, aggression and force are used to overwhelm whatever resistance is there.

Also because we live in a very competitive world, the attitude of win-lose is prevalent in relationships too. Culturally, many of us come from families where one parent is dominant and the other takes a more submissive or placating role. In these families, the emphasis is on doing things "right" (or "my way"); any other way is wrong. Therefore, there are blamers and the blamed; victims and victimizer. An either-or view of the world pervades these families. Unfortunately, there is no room for negotiating, for examining alternative possibilities, choices, or more importantly, for viewing each person's contributions as valid, appropriate and worthy of consideration.

There is another side of power. Webster defines power as "the ability or capacity to act or perform effectively." The Latin word for power (posse) means "to be able." In terms of marriage, each partner is viewed as having abilities or capacities to perform effectively in order to complete tasks and achieve goals.

Furthermore, establishing and maintaining a satisfactory relationship with respect to power includes: the decision-making process between the partners; their abilities to share responsibilities, manage finances, household tasks, child-rearing; and developing the structure by which they will accomplish these day-to-day activities. In addition, the couple must build boundaries that are flexible and expansive enough to permit testing and experimentation with new roles/positions that they each may take in relation to each other. Finally, the couple will need the skills to work through the many differences that they will discover about each other.

Besides capacities, abilities, skills and knowledge that each spouse brings into the relationship, power also includes self-realization and self-actualization within the context of marriage.

Needless to say, exerting power also results in conflicts. Many people view conflicts as something to be avoided at all costs; usually because in their families of origin, conflicts resulted in "yelling and screaming," "fights" (verbal, physical or both), and, generally, in a chaotic environment. Some couples go to the other extreme and respond to conflicts with silence, withdrawal, or compliance ("peace at any price"). The loss of Self is too high a price to pay and the Self is sacrificed in both the violent and the silent families.

An alternative way of looking at conflict is as a signal that there is something to be learned about Self and Other. Since people are different in many ways, couples can agree to view their differences and differentness as enhancing their relationship, rather than as threatening or rejecting.

GOALS OF THE THIRD STAGE

The goal, in terms of power, is to attain a balance of power between two people in an atmosphere of trust where each may express his/her own capacities, abilities and talents and where each is acknowledged and appreciated for his/her contributions in working together and in developing and maintaining a home that will be a haven for both people. To achieve this balance of power, the couple must be willing to perform the following tasks:

1. Expand the boundaries of the relationship so each partner will bring forth their hidden aspects into full view.
2. Reconcile their differences and polarization of their positions by accepting positive and negative traits of Self and Other.
3. Establish a foundation of support, empathy and connectedness by sharing the wounded aspects of their lives with each other.

SKILLS, ASSESSMENT INSTRUMENTS, AND INTERVENTIONS

The most common complaint that is heard from couples seeking help with troubled marriages is, "We cannot communicate." The basic tools that every couple needs to achieve a successful relationship, and which are an inherent part of therapy are: communication, problem-solving, conflict-resolution, negotiation and empathy-building skills.

Recent research (Gottman, 1994; Markman, 1994; Olson, 1990) is demonstrating that couples who have these skills can survive and feel more satisfied with their relationships. Markman (1994) of the University of Denver and Olson (1990) have found that the two major predictors of marital success are communication and conflict resolution. Gottman (1994), at the University of Washington in Seattle, studied 2,000 couples over two decades and concluded that the key to happiness "results from a couple's ability to resolve the conflicts that are inevitable in any relationship" (p. 28). Clinical observations and, now, empirical research are demonstrating that the belief that happy couples "never fight" is false. Markman (1994) states unequivocally, "One of the most powerful things you can do to protect your marriage is to learn constructive ways to handle conflict, differences, and disagreements" (p. 13).

Besides teaching couples the above skills (both in therapy and in classes), data-gathering and assessment instruments are necessary for better understanding:

1. Couple dynamics.
2. The influence of family backgrounds on the marital relationship.
3. The stage of development that each has mastered as individuals and as a couple, and
4. Where the couple is "stuck" in the process.

The major assessment-diagnostic instruments that have been found to be useful are The Family Genogram (McGoldrick, 1985), the Bader-Pearson Couple Diagnostic Questionnaire (1988), and the Prepare, Prepare-MC, and Enrich Inventories for pre-married, re-married and married couples (Olson, 1990).

The Family Genogram as a basic procedure used early in the therapy sessions provides the facts that enable the work to begin on the family of origin of each partner. Diagramming the families from the beginning presents the idea that each came from a family with a different structure and process, and to demonstrate how each was influenced by their parents' models of marriage. With this information made explicit, the couples have no basis for blaming or attacking each other. In effect, the genogram helps the couple shift the focus from faulting and blaming each other to a more objective position with each other and their problems.

Not only does the therapist derive objective data from the use of the genogram, but also multigenerational patterns become evident as well as providing information about critical and significant events, for example, births, deaths and other losses. It is also a valuable vehicle for disclosing triangular relationships, assumptions about roles (especially marital roles), rules that were operating in each family regarding relationships, communication, differentness, expression of emotions and for revealing the wounds that were not healed in early efforts toward separation-individuation.

At the same time the family genograms are being diagrammed, the therapist also gathers perceptual history data about the parents as husband/wife as well as mother/father. Whatever issue is presented as a problem of conflict between the pair has its roots in the family of origin. Whether the incident that triggered the emotionality is money, children, affection or an affair, the response is to go back to the family genogram to find the source: "How did you see your mother and father dealing with that issue?" In one instance, it was discovered that a husband's withdrawal in a three-year marriage was rooted in his unresolved grief over the loss of a father and sister who were killed in an accident when he was ten years old. In another relationship in which one was having an affair, the wife remembered that her mother was having an affair when she was six years old. In the couple therapy, she was able to confront the feelings from her childhood as well as dealing with the affair in her own life. Unresolved parental issues also get re-enacted in the marriages of adult children.

When the family perceptual history and the family genograms are used in conjunction with presenting problems, the spouses and the therapist recognize the different ways that each family of origin operated. Frequently, one or both spouses become so intrigued with family patterns that they turn their attention to exploring family dynamics with other family members.

The Marital History is also acquired in the early sessions from the spouses. Initially, while acquiring demographic information, the dates of any previous marriages should be recorded. This important information may be referred to in later sessions when examining repetitive patterns of conflict that may indicate unresolved areas from former relationships that also may be projected onto the present relationship.

Information about the courtship period and the characteristics that attracted them to each other may be reserved for the times when the therapist is confronted with hostile interactions between the couple. This information can be used to reframe the hostility and demonstrate to the couple that there was positive bonding that took place at another time. This rediscovery of the positive emotional resources (respect, caring, trust and love) that once bonded them are the essential ingredients for rebuilding and maintaining the relationship and encouraging growth.

The Bader-Pearson Couple Diagnostic Questionnaire (1988) is given to each spouse to fill out separately and to mail or bring to the next session. This is a more in-depth instrument that is useful in several ways:

1. In determining the stage of development that each partner has mastered.
2. As a means for each partner to openly express his/her thoughts, feeling and perceptions of the marital relationship.
3. As a stimulus for a live interactional exchange between the partners under the guidance and direction of the therapist.
4. In determining the "stuck" points (or impasses).

Now, for an example of an intervention–called Focusing–that is used whenever intense emotions are exhibited in the therapy session. The partner who is exhibiting the intense feelings is asked to describe in graphic terms (size, shape, color, texture) how s/he perceives the emotions and to pinpoint in the body where the emotions are located. The other partner observing is asked "to be there" to experience the feelings without attempting to rescue, avoid or suppress the emotions.

Then, the partner experiencing the emotions is asked to focus on the images or memories that may be evoked as s/he continues to focus. Frequently, the images or memories that surface are related to core issues that occurred in childhood or adolescence. With this technique clients have uncovered losses, abuse, neglect and many other painful early experiences that have remained unresolved and festering.

The uncovered core issues may require individual therapy; however, if both partners agree, we continue exploring and dealing with the core issue in the couple therapy sessions. Usually, an intense experience in one will re-awaken early painful experiences in the other. Even more importantly, sharing painful experiences with each other opens the way for growing empathy and understanding between the two partners.

HELPFUL HINTS FOR COUPLES

1. When you feel stuck and do not know how to proceed, go back into your memory and remember family interactions. The key is there. This is not to blame parents. More importantly, this is an opportunity to discover *how* family interactions influenced the behavior manifested in your present relationship.
2. *Marital struggles are unfinished business with parents or battles observed between parents.* In the family, patterns of behavior are learned as ways of coping with stresses. In marriage, scenes from the family are re-enacted over and over in an effort to resolve or complete what was left unfinished from childhood.
3. Projection is the mechanism by which we see in the partner the unacceptable behaviors that were experienced in the family of origin.
4. The process of separating the present problem from the original wound takes time, patience and tender loving care for your Self and your partner.
5. It is crucial in dealing with power struggles that you stay focused on and connected to your partner in the present and rediscover that person whenever you lose touch with him/her.
6. Responding to each other's pain with empathy and understanding and nurturing each other in the relationship is vital for the growth of intimacy between you.

SUMMARY

In the third stage of marriage, the couple is confronted with one of the most difficult and critical issues in marriage—power. The customary definitions of power lead to distancing, polarization and erosion of the relationship.

Another view of power has been presented. In this view of power, self-assertion, within the context of marriage, permits the couple to confront their conflicts in more effective ways. Approaching conflicts as opportunities for learning and growth, the therapist guides the couple toward completing their "unfinished business" with parents and family of origin, expanding the boundaries of marriage to include their vulnerabilities, appreciating and accepting their differences and differentness and, most importantly, laying a more empathetic foundation for an intimate relationship.

REFERENCES

Bader, E. and Pearson, P. (1988). *In Quest of the Mythical Mate. A Developmental Approach to Diagnosis and Treatment in Couples Therapy.* New York: Brunner/Mazel Publishers, 231-232.

Gottman, J. and Silver, N. (1994). *Why Marriages Succeed or Fail.* New York: Simon and Schuster.

Hendrix, H. (1988). *Getting the Love You Want. A Guide for Couples.* New York: Henry Holt and Co.

Kovacs, L. (1988). Couple Therapy: An Integrated Developmental and Family Systems Model. *Family Therapy,* 15, (2), 132-155.

Markman, H., Stanley, S., Blumberg, S.L. (1994). *Fighting for Your Marriage.* San Francisco: Jossey-Bass, Inc. Publishers.

May, R. (1972). *Power and Innocence.* New York: W.W. Norton and Co., Inc., p. 20.

McGoldrich, M. and Gerson, R. (1985). *Genograms in Family Assessment.* New York: W.W. Norton and Co., Inc.

Napier, A. with Whitaker, C.A. (1978). *The Family Crucible.* New York: Harper and Row Publishers.

Olson, D.G. (1990). Marriage in Perspective. In Fincham, F.D. and Bradbury, T.N., Editors. *The Psychology of Marriage. Basic Issues and Application.* New York: The Guilford Press.

Satir, V. (1964). *Conjoint Family Therapy. A Guide to Theory and Technique.* Palo Alto, CA: Science and Behavior Books, Inc.

Travers, J.A. Love and Marriage and Other Silly Delusions. *Journal of Couples Therapy,* 2 (3), p. 86.

Dependency and Counter-Dependency in Couples

Terry A. Kupers

SUMMARY. There is a tendency on the part of many men in couples to deny their dependency needs, and for the women in these couples to view themselves as excessively needy. These uneven subjective perceptions are examined, as are the ways contemporary gender socialization interferes with the attainment of the ideal of mutual dependency in couples. Some implications for couples therapy are explored. *[Article copies available for a fee from The Haworth Document Delivery Service: 1-800-342-9678. E-mail address: getinfo@haworth.com]*

A man leaves his wife of nine years. The identifiable impetus is his attraction to another woman, a "more independent and exciting" woman who lives by herself and seems always available to try new things and strike out on new adventures. In comparison, his wife seems "clingy and dependent." After leaving his wife he gets involved with the "more exciting" woman. Shortly thereafter he begins to feel very alone. He does not think the new relationship is working. His new romantic interest is very attentive to him, and exciting, when they are together, but she is also involved with other men and other activities that do not include him. He feels jealous, threatened and unloved. He begins to consider going back to his wife.

Meanwhile, after suffering a massive depression following the deser-

---

Terry A. Kupers, MD, teaches at The Wright Institute, Berkeley, Oakland, CA 94610.

[Haworth co-indexing entry note]: "Dependency and Counter-Dependency in Couples." Kupers, Terry A. Co-published simultaneously in *Journal of Couples Therapy* (The Haworth Press, Inc.) Vol. 7, No. 1, 1997, pp. 39-47; and: *When One Partner Is Willing and the Other Is Not* (ed: Barbara Jo Brothers) The Haworth Press, Inc., 1997, pp. 39-47. Single or multiple copies of this article are available for a fee from The Haworth Document Delivery Service [1-800-342-9678, 9:00 a.m. - 5:00 p.m. (EST). E-mail address: getinfo@haworth.com].

tion by her husband, the man's wife begins to put her life back together. She develops new friendships and takes part in new activities. She realizes she never did these things while she was married because she felt too dependent on her husband. Or was she so dependent? In therapy she begins to figure out that what she believed to be her dependency included a certain amount of duty, the "wifely duty" to be available and attentive to her husband at all times. In other words, for all the years she was married she kept convincing herself that she was the only one who was dependent, and that belief kept her from forming the kinds of friendships and partaking in the kinds of activities that might make her unavailable when her husband needed to have her around.

After a few months of separation, he breaks off his new relationship, falls into a depression, and approaches his wife to see if she would be interested in trying to get back together. She is no longer depressed and is enjoying her new, more "independent" life. She is very angry at her husband for leaving her for another woman and for making her believe she is the clingy one. But she also realizes she still loves him. So, following the advice of her individual therapist, she tells him she would consider talking about reconciliation, but only in the presence of a couples therapist. In the first session of couples therapy he admits that it was only after he left his wife, thinking of her as clingy and dependent, that he realized that he was quite dependent on being depended upon by her. She cries for several minutes. Then she summons the breath to tell him that it was only after he left her, and she got over feeling devastated and uncertain she wanted to go on with her life, that she realized she was quite capable of being more independent. Something about their marriage made her feel like she was the dependent one, and made him feel like the only way he could be free of excessive dependency was to leave her. The couple proceeds to negotiate a reconciliation–but on entirely new terms, including the establishment of a mature, and consensually recognized mutual dependency.

The unevenness in this couple is about dependency and its denial (i.e., counter-dependency). Gender socialization plays a large part, since counter-dependency is typically a male trait in this culture. However, there are quite a few straight couples–a sizable minority–wherein the gender roles are reversed and it is the woman who is compelled, perhaps unconsciously, to deny her dependency needs, while the man is more open to expressing his dependency needs–but he feels bad that his appreciation for her taking such good care of him is not reciprocated. Or, in gay and lesbian relationships, dependency and counter-dependency might also be unevenly distributed between the partners. In each case, this kind of unevenness can become an important issue in couples therapy.

DEPENDENCY, A SUBJECTIVE PHENOMENON

If the definition of dependency is limited to financial matters, it is possible to decide objectively who in a couple is more dependent upon whom. Thus, if a husband works and a wife stays home and takes care of the children, it is apparent that she is (financially) dependent on him. If he is disabled, or she continues to work while he is unemployed, the roles are reversed. But as soon as the definition of dependency is expanded, for instance to include the satisfaction of emotional needs, the picture becomes much more complicated. Even in the case where the man is the sole provider for the family, if he, like the average American male, were almost exclusively dependent on his female partner for emotional connection and sustenance, and also needed her to provide the nurturing environment for his children to grow up healthily, then it would be much more difficult to decide who was more or less dependent on whom. Is she more dependent on him because he provides financially for her and the children, or is he the more dependent one because without her he would starve emotionally and be incapable of relating very well with his children? As soon as dependency is defined at all broadly, it becomes a matter of subjective interpretation.

Even if the situation is too complicated to permit objective appraisal, there might still be consensus within the couple about who is more dependent on whom. For instance, it is possible for a husband and wife to share the view that she is clingy and dependent while he is much more independent—whether or not the unevenness can be objectively substantiated. Or, the partners might disagree strongly about who is more dependent. Thus, many women, influenced by feminist discussions of recent decades, have been standing up to their partners and pointing out that a man's exclusive dependence on a woman partner for emotional sustenance makes it hard for the woman to develop independent friends and interests—perhaps it would be better if he looked for some same-sex friends and interests independent of her so she could be free to have her independent pursuits. The point comes as a revelation to many men who had previously believed that their female partners were the dependent ones.

By having this kind of dialogue, couples are broadening the definition of dependency and struggling to arrive at a new consensus about a subjective phenomenon. The key term is struggle. When a couple is capable of struggling in an open and principled way about such issues, and each is willing to admit the ways he or she has been colluding in a distorted view of the dependency that exists between them, a new consensus emerges and there is little need for couples therapy.

An outsider's perception of how dependency works within a couple might be quite different than that of either partner. Thus, when one of the partners confides in a friend that he or she feels like the clingy one in the relationship, the friend might disagree. Thus, a woman might tell a friend that she feels like a nag because she is the only one who worries about a child's difficulties in school while her husband always says things will work out fine; only to hear from her friend that it is her husband who is the needy one—he needs her to keep track of the child's problems so his mind can be free to deal with work-related issues. Or, a man who believes he is useless around the house and his wife is the one who always takes care of the children, is reminded by a male friend about the many meals he cooks on weekends, the fact that he does all the gardening and repairs, and that he is very involved in his kids' soccer teams. In other words, the dependency that exists within a couple might be viewed somewhat more objectively by someone outside the couple who does not share the partners' collusive need to maintain a particular subjective perception about their relationship. Couples therapists can use their perceptions as outsiders to help couples demystify their perceptions about who is dependent upon whom, and for what.

MUTUAL DEPENDENCY

In couples who remain together for any significant length of time, dependency is usually quite mutual, even in cases where it appears very uni-directional. Thus, in the clinical vignette that opens this article, the husband and wife were each dependent on the other, but they created a shared illusion that she was the dependent one while he was quite independent. It was only after they split up that he discovered he had always been dependent on being depended upon. This is frequently the pattern in couples where the dependency at first seems most extreme and unilateral. For instance, consider the couple where the wife is physically ill, suffers from severe social phobia or is very depressed. It might seem to an outsider that the husband is the strong, independent one who is always running around frantically caring for a sick, dependent wife; but in reality there must be a shared need on the part of the partners to maintain that impression. The couples therapist has the difficult task of figuring out and helping the couple understand exactly why both partners need to view the relationship as so lopsidedly dependent, and how they both collude in keeping it so.

Fairbairn (1952) contrasts infantile and mature dependence. Infantile dependence involves severe separation anxiety that keeps the child (or the childlike adult) dependent on the object (originally the mother) with whom he or she is merged. Mature dependence, on the other hand, "is characterized by a capacity on the part of a differentiated individual for co-operative relationships with differentiated objects" (Fairbairn, 1952, p. 145). Notice that, for Fairbairn, the goal is not "independence," it is "mutual dependence," which he characterizes as "a relationship involving evenly matched giving and taking between two differentiated individuals who are mutually dependent, and between whom there is no disparity of dependence" (Ibid.).

Dicks (1967) carries Fairbairn's formulation into couples therapy, pointing out that it is the projective identifications of both partners that obstruct the evolution and recognition of mutual dependence. An example would be the man who cannot tolerate any sign of dependency in himself, projects all dependency needs onto his female partner, and then behaves toward her in ways that cause her to act out his projections. For instance, he might infantilize her and do so much for her in the name of husbandly caretaking that she begins to feel she is incapable of doing anything for herself. The woman who colludes in acting out her partner's projective identification has an unconscious need to project reciprocal unacceptable qualities. For instance, she might dread separation and loss so much, and believe her father's warning that if she is too strong and independent she will lose her man, that she feels a need to project the image of the independent person onto her male partner. The partners share the illusion that she is the only one who has dependency needs.

THE GENDERED MISRECOGNITION OF DEPENDENCY IN COUPLES

It is not accidental that more often than not the woman is viewed as the dependent one, and the man as the more independent one who takes care of her. Where this stereotype is at play the man's emotional dependence on the woman is generally ignored—but this is no accident, either. Beliefs about dependency are shaped to a significant extent by our gender biases. When feminists demand recognition for women for the work they do at home, they are blowing the whistle on the stereotypic unevenness that permitted men, most of whom were almost entirely dependent on their female partners for emotional sustenance, to claim that it was the women, and not them, who were the dependent ones.

The denial of dependency, or "counter-dependency," is part of the "normal" male make-up. Boys are told not to cry when they are hurt lest they be considered "sissies," and thus they are trained in a rigid kind of self-sufficiency. If they were to cry, for instance after sustaining an injury during an athletic event, and were to seek a hug from a supportive adult, they would be exhibiting emotional dependency. That is precisely what they are taught to avoid. In fact, as both women and men writing about gender issues have pointed out, males in our society are socialized to be counter-dependent (Osherson, 1992, & Rubin, 1983). Besides being taught not to cry, they are trained to keep their cards close to their chest, act self-sufficiently, not to let the other guy know when they are hurt, not to be a "Mommy's boy" and so forth. Girls, on the other hand, are permitted to express their feelings, and to respond empathically to the feelings of others, as if all that is part of their training to be wives and mothers. In other words, while male children are socialized to be counter-dependent, female children are socialized to be forthcoming about their emotional dependency, and to seek the emotional support of others.

There is a striking exception to this kind of rigid role socialization. It is permissible for men, even "real men," to cry and seek emotional support from their female partners. This does not make them "sissies" or "weaklings." But if they were to be that way with other men, especially at work or in public, they would be viewed as less than manly. So men tend to develop an exclusive emotional dependency, and often an unusual openness, with their female partners. But there are some limitations in the permission the reigning male culture grants them in this regard. They are not supposed to let others see that they are this emotionally open and vulnerable with anyone, so when a female partner tells one of her women friends about her mate's weaknesses and self-doubts, and the man finds out his partner has exposed him in this way, he is likely to get very angry at her for airing his dirty laundry in public.

In addition, even inside the couple where it is acceptable for the man to be emotionally dependent, nothing is to be said about his dependency. Thus it is not uncommon for a man to be very needy with his wife, but get very upset if she ever explicitly mentions the extent of his neediness. Women, as part of their socialization, learn to avoid mentioning their male partner's neediness. And by not mentioning it, they are in effect taking care of his unstated needs, but getting no recognition for it.

Even as gender roles change, some of this kind of traditional socialization survives. For instance, in the workplace, men and women, on average, tend to function in different manners. Men are more likely to work independently on a problem or a task, find a solution or complete a project, and then expect credit for doing so. Women are more likely to work collaboratively with other women in the workplace, even if this simply means brainstorming together before attempting a task, and then to share the credit. Of course this is a huge generalization, and there are many exceptions in both directions. And, as women move higher up in previously all-male hierarchies at work and challenge the glass ceiling, it may turn out that they have to adopt male ways of working. But this gendered difference in the way work is carried out serves as one more illustration of the way women tend to admit their dependence on others while men try to hide it.

Feminists at the Stone Center at Wellesley College point out that official psychiatry as well as many psychotherapists have incorporated this society's gender biases in drawing lines between normal and pathological qualities, and in deciding which material to interpret in psychotherapy (Jordan et al., 1991). Generally, women's need for connection is pathologized, or interpreted as an expression of insufficient autonomy, while men's obsessive need to be independent and not reliant on anyone, as well as men's hesitation to form close same-sex friendships wherein mutual dependency might develop, are left uninterpreted. This kind of gender bias is reflected in DSM-IV. For instance, while the diagnosis Dependent Personality Disorder is assigned disproportionately to women, there is no equivalent diagnostic category for men who dread intimacy and dependency (Kupers, 1995).

Returning to the way couples present in therapy, the continuing uneven recognition of dependency can create a therapeutic impasse. Perhaps the man refuses to move past the notion that the woman is clingy and emotionally demanding. Or, when it comes to light during a couples therapy session that the man is at least equally dependent in some previously unrecognized regard, he might become incensed with his partner after the session for having exposed him so humiliatingly in front of another person (the therapist). If the couples therapist does not detect this drama-in-the-making and intervene during the session, perhaps by giving the man a chance to say he is angry about the unfair treatment he believes he is receiving, the couple might even terminate the treatment prior to the next appointment.

COUPLES THERAPY AND THE ATTAINMENT OF MUTUAL DEPENDENCY

This is not to say men are more likely than women to resort to denial in couples or in couples therapy. Probably the amount of denial by men and women is approximately equal (and opposite), but it is generally about different issues. For instance, where there is denial of dependency on the part of the man, there might be denial of independence on the part of his female partner–out of fear that her independence will be the cause of his leaving. However, on the issue of dependency, men are more likely to deny theirs, and this is a matter of gender role socialization, not insincerity or malevolence. It is very difficult to be a man in this society and readily admit one's dependencies. This is one reason why men whose female partners make more money than they do, or inherit more, are so prone to feel shame about their relative financial dependency. It is also why men have so much trouble accepting the status of disabled. When a man is an able provider and brings more money into the relationship, something seems as it ought to be, according to an all-too-familiar tradition.

But this is precisely why the man's counter-dependency, once it is openly recognized, provides such a wonderful opportunity for a break-through in couples therapy. The refusal to admit dependency is a central requirement of traditional masculinity, so when a woman or a couples therapist confronts a man about this, and the man is willing to struggle to transcend his denial, the couple has a rare opportunity to re-examine the gender assumptions that underlie their relationship, and to consciously opt to transform some of their unspoken assumptions and habits (Kupers, 1993).

The easiest application of this formulation is the case where the couple is very open to this kind of insight, is relieved to have their previously inexplicable discord explained to them in this fashion, have enough love for one another to work hard in couples therapy, and readily set out to re-examine and re-arrange their gendered relationship. Many couples therapies do not proceed this smoothly. Many times the therapist is alone in detecting the man's counter-dependency and the woman's efforts to protect her partner's self-image by viewing herself as the clingy one. In other words, the couple rejects the interpretation. Or perhaps the woman joins the therapist in seeing the pattern, but the man continues to deny it, leaving the woman with the choice of continuing to confront her mate until he feels that she and the therapist are teaming up on him and he sabotages the therapy, or to disregard the insight she has gained from the couples therapy and to continue playing along with her mate's counter-dependency.

The therapist must be tactful and artful as he or she helps both members of the couple feel they are getting a fair hearing so they can eventually move past the stuck place of collusive denial and defensiveness. The test of the success of the couples therapy is whether the two individuals feel that the struggle they have engaged in as a couple to recognize and acknowledge their mutual dependency carries over to their lives as individuals, and that they are each better people for it.

REFERENCES

Dicks, H.V. (1967). *Marital tensions*. New York: Basic Books.

Fairbairn, W.R. (1952). *Psychoanalytic studies of the personality: The object relation theory of personality*. London: Tavistock Publications.

Jordan, J., Kaplan, A., Miller, J.B., Stiver, I.P., and Surrey, J.L. (1991). *Women's growth in connection: Writings from the Stone Center*. New York: Guilford Press.

Kupers, T. (1993). *Revisioning men's lives: Gender, intimacy and power*. New York: Guilford Press.

Kupers, T. (1995). The politics of psychiatry: Gender and sexual preference in DSM-IV. *Masculinities*, 3,2, 1-12.

Osherson, S. (1992). *Wrestling with love: How men struggle with intimacy with women, children, parents, and each other*. New York: Fawcett Columbine.

Rubin, L. (1983). *Intimate strangers: Men and women together*. New York: Harper Colophon Books.

The Cycle of Violence:
An Integrative Clinical Approach

George J. Steinfeld

SUMMARY. An integrative clinical model is described, entitled TARET Systems. This model has been applied in the treatment of male batterers and their partners. This paper applies the approach to an expanded version of the cycle of violence from three to four stages. A rationale for therapeutic interventions is presented for each stage utilizing a brief, solution focused approach within the broader cognitive-behavioral systems stress framework. Professional dilemmas are discussed throughout the paper. *[Article copies available for a fee from The Haworth Document Delivery Service: 1-800-342-9678. E-mail address: getinfo@haworth.com]*

The focus of this paper will be the author's clinical approach to the cycle of violence (COV) (Walker, 1979, 1984; Deschner, 1984). Clinical experience attests to the reality of this interactional pattern in violent couples, and research (Walker, 1984) has supported the general concept. The purpose of this paper will be to expand the cycle of violence from a three to a four stage model, and to suggest ways of intervening with an individual or couple to break the destructive pattern in the current relationship, and to stop the inter-generational transmission process from continuing. A previous paper described the author's general clinical model with abusive individuals and couples (Steinfeld, 1989). Here, he will zero in on

George J. Steinfeld, PhD, is Director, Center for Brief Psychotherapy, 1145 Daniels Farm Road, Trumbull, CT 06611.

[Haworth co-indexing entry note]: "The Cycle of Violence: An Integrative Clinical Approach." Steinfeld, George J. Co-published simultaneously in *Journal of Couples Therapy* (The Haworth Press, Inc.) Vol. 7, No. 1, 1997, pp. 49-81; and: *When One Partner Is Willing and the Other Is Not* (ed: Barbara Jo Brothers) The Haworth Press, Inc., 1997, pp. 49-81. Single or multiple copies of this article are available for a fee from The Haworth Document Delivery Service [1-800-342-9678, 9:00 a.m. - 5:00 p.m. (EST). E-mail address: getinfo@haworth.com].

49

the specifics of the violent cycle from an integrative perspective. By integrative I mean a cognitive-behavioral-systems approach within a solution focused framework, which can be used with individuals or couples.

Though the cycle of violence can be described and experienced, description is not explanation, and, in describing a pattern it is not always easy to determine a beginning, a middle and an end. Who does what to whom, how, when, under what circumstances, and for what reasons, is a function of the observers, in and out of the interactional system. Therefore, although couples, therapists and researchers can agree that a pattern exists (consensual validation), agreement does not make something ultimately "true" (witness the tyranny of any group). Why the pattern exists, and what to do to break a destructive pattern is still being debated.

All ongoing couple relationships are punctuated by conflict. In working with couples where there has been physical, mental and emotional abuse, clinicians and clients need a framework within which to understand and eventually help change these destructive patterns. The author employs an interactional, stress framework, and a cognitive-constructivist-systems perspective to help individuals and couples break the cycle of violence, and substitute more adaptive patterns of behavior. What adaptive means is a negotiable pattern, to be defined and contracted for by the client (individual or couple) and the provider (who is constrained by the law and his/her personal values and viewpoint regarding power and control issues in human relationships). The levels of work, both personal and interpersonal, which can be focused on has been described in a previous paper (Steinfeld, 1989) and will be noted later. By focusing on an in-depth analysis of the four stages of the COV, and interventions which help clients deepen their understanding of their respective reactions, we hope to reach our goals of eliminating violence and reducing destructive conflict. Instead, we hope to facilitate more cooperation, collaboration, compromise, compassion and commitment, as well as more intimacy in their relationship. Recent clinical theory and research (Baucom, 1995) suggests that there are F.A.C.T.s about long term relationships that therapists can foster in couples (Forgiveness, Acceptance, Commitment, Trust).

STRESS AND FAMILY VIOLENCE

Farrington (1986) investigated the relationship between social stress and family violence. "Stress can be said to be present within an individual or social system to the extent that there exists a discrepancy between the demand posed by the stressor (including either or both objective and subjective demand) and the coping behaviors drawn from the individual's or social system's response capabilities. . . . [The] system can be said to be under stress if, for any of a variety of reasons, the response offered in the face of the stressor stimulus is not sufficient to adequately minimize or otherwise negate the demand generated by the stimulus" (p. 133). This definition is very close to the one offered by Novaco (1979) and employed here, along with the clinical theories.

Unlike Farrington's work, however, this article relates stress concepts to the specifics of the cycle of violence in couples. By focusing on the interactional pattern of violence, therapists and clients may be able to obtain a clearer grasp of the stressors (physical, environmental, physiological, psychological, social). We can help couples understand the cognitive-emotional-behavioral consequences for the persons involved. By so doing, cognitive-behavioral changes can be facilitated which would negate these stressors and/or help clients cope effectively with them.

In choosing my approach to the cycle of violence with couples, the writer decided to place the main emphasis on the perpetrator of the abuse. Although it had previously been thought that men are overwhelmingly the perpetrators of abuse, recent evidence suggests that levels of abuse in couples are about equal for men and women, but that male violence is considerably more damaging. Further, "spousal aggression often starts early in a dating relationship and, for perhaps as many as 25-30% of those who report first instances of aggression in early dating relationships, it escalates to more severe forms across time" (O'Leary & Cascardi, 1996). My decision to focus primarily, but not exclusively, on the man is based on the underlying assumption, and belief, backed by empirical data and research, that the abuser has a problem with self control (among other problems), and that no matter what the woman may or may not have done, which he "perceived" as a provocation, he is responsible for his abusive behavior. The woman's role in the escalation of the couple's conflictual relationship may also be confronted (in individual and couple's therapy), although the focus is still on the man's aggressive behavior, which needs to be understood and changed. This position is consistent with a cognitive-behavioral-systems model, whereby aggressive behavior is thought to be learned, and can, therefore, be unlearned. This position also allows for the integration of the feminist and family systems perspectives in the treatment of domestic violence. The integration of the cognitive-behavioral and family systems (interactional) models has been spelled out elsewhere (Steinfeld, 1980; 1989). A feminist critique of family systems theory in relation to family violence has been addressed (Bograd, 1984). Dell (1989) has also discussed the issue of power and control from a family systems perspective. Virginia Goldner has spoken about the problem of family violence from a gender perspective (at various meetings of the American Family Therapy Association). She and her colleagues at the Ackerman Institute have developed a model for dealing with abuse in couples (Goldner, Penn, Scheinberg & Walker, 1990). The writer's approach addresses many of the points made by feminist theorist-practitioners who are aware and sensitive to the unequal power relationships that exist in families.

We have not discussed the nature of power in male-female relationships. Clinically, however, or from an experiential perspective, that is, from inside the skin of men and women, the latter perceive themselves as less physically powerful than men. Men, most often, but not always, agree. Psychologically, however, who has more power in the relationship is debatable. We hear different perspectives based on who is describing the nature of the specific conflict or relationship issue. This observation comes from more than 25 years of work with individuals and couples, and directing a batterer's group in Connecticut for almost ten years (Men & Stress Control, YMCA, Bridgeport). From the man's point of view, his physical abuse is motivated by a host of factors, not the least of which is his "perceived" need to feel powerful in a relationship in which he experiences himself to feel insecure and "needy." Men often feel intimidated by their wives (and their verbal and other abilities), while denying their own intimidating actions and tendencies. The inability to perceive one's role as a perpetrator, or in generating just those behaviors in others that one perceives as a provocative stressor, is common in most conflicting couples and especially evident in male batterers. Instead, the male perpetrator perceives his behavior as existing independent of his actions, or the context. This tendency to see oneself as a "reactor" to external events is very common in conflicting couples, and in emotionally immature persons in general is conceived by this writer to be a function of a "cognitive deficit," namely, one's egocentricity, a primitive, or less developed stage of cognitive development (Piaget, 1962; Feffer, 1970). A male batterer's egocentricity, neediness, personal insecurity in many aspects of his life (Dutton, 1995), and sense of entitlement in his home, has led to his abusive behavior. This is his illegal and dysfunctional attempt to gain or regain some sense of power and control over a person and relationship that he feels he deserves and feels he needs to feel like a "man," as the above research has described. But complex motivations cannot be used as an excuse, so that the focus of therapy is to help the batterer gain more power and control over himself, or those aspects of his perceived self that he experiences as "helpless and powerless," not only in his relationship with his female partner, but in other aspects of his life as well. Several of the ideas relating to gender role issues will be integrated into the current clinical work with violent men and couples.

COGNITIVE-BEHAVIORAL-SYSTEMS: INTEGRATED, PROCESS ORIENTED THERAPY

At this point we will move into the clinical material. The therapy model employed by the author will be outlined briefly, since a more extensive description can be found in previous papers (1980; 1989). Whereas the earlier monograph described the theoretical and spiritual framework, the later paper applied the clinical approach to spouse abuse.

INTERACTIONAL STRESS MODEL IN RELATION TO THE CYCLE OF VIOLENCE

In an early paper (1975), the writer presented a theoretical basis for a specific mode of cognitive therapy, namely, Rational Emotive psychotherapy (RET). RET, as a cognitive therapy, stems from a theory of form perception (Zuckerman & Rock, 1957). This cognitive theory of form perception has been extended to interpersonal perception, and is continuing to evolve into an integrative, constructivist approach to therapy (Steinfeld, *in preparation*). A cognitive approach to form perception makes the following distinctions:

a. the stimulus, which refers to an activating event which can be described geometrically, or as a video tape recorder would show events, or as a Zen master would describe events;
b. the interpretation of the stimulus, its cognitive meaning to the perceiver;
c. the response to the stimulus, its verbal, linguistic label, or the physiological and behavioral response.

The response, as will be described and elaborated, is a function of a number of factors:

a. the perceptual process, the awareness of the event, and the interpretation or meaning of that stimulus;
b. the feeling attached to that meaning or interpretation of that stimulus;
c. the anticipated (in thought) consequences, and actual history of the consequences of one's actions, as conditioned by past experience and/or constrained by a limited response repertoire.

Cognitive aspects of meaning have to do with thoughts, in terms of language and images, assumptions, expectations, attribution, standards, and values. These cognitions may be "rational" or "irrational" (Ellis, 1962). A more useful framework for evaluating cognitions is for the client to determine if they are functional or dysfunctional, in terms of their outcome (their emotional and behavioral consequences). "Do these cognitions, and the feelings and behaviors which flow from them, get you what you want in the short and long run, or are they dysfunctional (lead to affective and behavioral consequences which interfere with getting what you want and need)?" In the latter case, the response would perpetuate negative cycles, which is the essence of an addictive process (Steinfeld, 1975).

The model to be described has been called TARET SYSTEMS (Steinfeld, 1980), and is a process oriented therapy. The name is less important than what it means, and how it is applied. It is basically a perceptual-learning model, relying heavily on a cognitive theory of perception, the laws of classical and instrumental conditioning, social learning theory, the clinical theories of Transactional Analysis, the cognitive theories of Ellis, Beck and other cognitive-behavior therapists, family systems theories, a constructivist philosophy, and Eastern spiritual perspectives. The model outlined below in its basic format, and how it is applied to stress related work, adapts the ABCs from Ellis, and "Personality," represented by the Parent, Adult and Child ego states of Berne (1961).

Ego state is a concept developed by Berne to represent a consistent pattern of thought, feeling and behavior. In general, however, the concept of "personality" is not given much consideration in this approach. "Personality" as a theoretical discipline may be useful in theory and research. But my experience (biased as it may be) indicates that it tends to obscure rather than clarify the nature of human experience, and how to relieve suffering. More frequently, personality categories, which started out describing a pattern of thought and behavior, are then "reified," and used to explain the behavior in question. This circular kind of thinking confuses people in their efforts to understand themselves and their dilemmas. Further, personality labels are often used to excuse dysfunctional behavior, e.g., I did this because I'm schizophrenic, or manic depressive, or alcoholic, or borderline, etc. This game of "wooden leg," described by Berne (1964), tends to keep clients from accepting responsibility for their lives, and is especially relevant to men who batter women.

The writer's experience, and that of every colleague he has met who has worked with batterers, confirms the observation that these men tend to blame the woman for their actions, or something else (e.g., alcohol, the kids, my past, I'm out of work, etc.) other than themselves. As discussed elsewhere (1989), this is one of the first and most important issues that need to be addressed when working with men who abuse women. But this is a general clinical issue with anyone who uses anger to intimidate and manipulate relationships. In the current model and clinical approach, anger is differentiated from the response to the self generated emotion (feelings are separated from the action, and the thought that generates both). As difficult as it is to get men to accept responsibility for their actions, it is even more difficult for them to see (understand) that they have generated their own anger. How this is done will be described later, and has been addressed in an earlier paper, just as it has been by other cognitive therapists. Not only is it difficult for violent men to accept responsibility for their feelings and actions, but almost all clients with whom the writer has worked have this problem of believing that they have generated their own feelings. When clients ultimately understand and accept this idea, therapy is nearing termination.

Finally, in the clinical model outlined below, the "witness" is a concept discussed by Ram Dass (1976), and other spiritual leaders, and one that the writer has found useful in clinical work. It represents the "higher self," what might be called the "super Adult," or the integrated self, or any other name we might give to the non-judgmental observer in all of us.

The TARET SYSTEMS model, as a cognitive-behavioral interactional approach, has been spelled out (Steinfeld, 1980). It has been used to describe an approach to family violence in general (1989). In this paper, the cycle of violence will be addressed using this process oriented model. The "hypothetical" cycle, yet "real" interactional pattern, will be described in detail as we proceed. As clinicians listen to couples describe their experiences, and what has happened to "cause" the violent episodes, how they have tried to increase or decrease the probability of their occurrence, and how they hope to decrease it in the future, or prevent it from ever happening again, this model offers them a framework within which to understand and break the pattern. Whereas more general clinical strategies have been spelled out in previous papers, some more specifics will be mentioned here.

STAGE 1: THE STAGE OF CALMNESS

At time one (T1), prior to the manifestation of problematic behavior (in our case, anger and the abusive behavior that accompanies this emotional response), the marital relationship exists whereby adaptive (constructive alternative) exchanges between the spouses are in the foreground. Emotional closeness is within tolerable limits, stress from within and without of the system is manageable, and the couple is in stage 1 of the cycle of violence. Regulation of emotional distance (whether learned in one's family of origin or elsewhere, or innate) is a core assumption of this model. Stress is a notion that plays a role in the couple's dance of intimacy, as does their assumptions about gender, power and control between men and women in close relationships. The complexities of these issues, as they are manifested in violent couples, is not the main focus of this paper. The hypothesis about Stage 1 is that the couple is emotionally close during this period of relative calm, and testimony from our cases gives this hypothesis clinical validity.

During this stage, each person's cognitive-affective-behavioral response tendencies are operating adaptively. Each spouse has appropriate expectations regarding their respective abilities to cope with the demands being made by themselves or the other. Stress is within tolerable limits. Since this is a vital stage to which the troubled couple wants to return, it is important to play close attention to what is happening during this time so that the couple can do more of it. Traditionally, clinicians have focused more on the problem area than on what is going well between the couple. In our approach, instead of focusing on the dysfunctional aspects of the relationship, the therapist can pay attention to this stage where calmness and closeness are comfortable for each partner.

The following questions are geared toward helping the couple to understand and foster this stage of calm and intimacy that can exist. It refocuses them from concerns about conflict and violence to more healthy and positive aspects of their relationship. Thus, in addition to asking about how the couple first came together, what attracted them, what kept them interested, and similar questions that many therapists employ, the current approach follows the brief treatment model of DeShazer (1982), M.R.I. Watzlawick et al., 1974, and others (O'hanlon, 1987; Weiner-Davis) by searching for solutions rather than problems:

A. Present Relationship

  1. When you're not arguing/fighting, what is happening that you want to continue to happen? If the couple or any member cannot describe what is happening under these conditions, the therapist can give them the First Session task to monitor their positive behavior and report back next session.
  2. When are you less likely to fight?
  3. Who is around when you don't fight?

4. On a scale from 1-10, when you're not fighting, how close do you feel to one another.
5. How close do you want to feel?
6. What stressors (upsetting things) are not happening when you are close?
7. What kinds of things do you find relaxing?
8. When does an argument not lead to violence? (search for anything that helps the perpetrator realize that he has control over his behavior, Steinfeld, 1989).
9. When is sex (love making) better–before, during, or after your fights (search for sex as a stimulus or reinforcing event associated with violence). In what ways is it better?
10. Who is most likely to feel comfortable when you're not fighting?

B. To help focus on reinforcing exchanges in their relationship ask questions having to do with when they are feeling good about themselves and the relationship, their attractive qualities, shared positive experiences of the past and present, etc.

C. To help with generational issues associated with the positive aspects of their relationship that exists in Stage 1: (Focusing on family of origin relationships helps some clients realize that much of their behavior has been learned through the modeling process, and can be unlearned through active re-decision making. It also explains things to clients and gives them hope that change can occur.)

1. In thinking about your parents' relationship, which one was most comfortable (uncomfortable) with closeness (distance)?
2. How would calm or closeness (intimacy) be expressed in your family of origin (between your parents).
3. How did you feel when your parents were getting along?
4. How do you think your children feel when you are close? How do they show it? How do you feel when they feel good about you?

D. Interventions between sessions to keep the focus on Stage 1:

1. General: Write down the kind of close loving relationship you want to have if a miracle happened overnight. Be specific so that we will all know when we have achieved our goals in therapy.
2. Any questions that foster a relationship vision that the couple can share.
3. First session task:

Pay attention to what you do when you overcome your urge to fight (argue, distance, etc. (De Shazer, 1988)).

Pay attention to what makes you feel good and close to your partner. Specifically, when do you feel most loved (loving)?

How are you able to let each other know when you appreciate each other; feel good about each other; compliment each other. How does it feel to do this? How come?

In what ways that you take each other for granted do you want to change?

Think about what pleases you and your partner so that we can discuss it at our next session.

Each of these above questions and the suggestions below are geared toward opening up possibilities to explore ways of enhancing Stage 1.

4. Pre-treatment changes: From the time you called to schedule an appointment to today, have you noticed any changes that you want to have more of?

5. Wiser-older self: Think about yourself as an older wiser person of about 80 or so years of age. What would the older wiser you say to you and your partner that might help in getting you to feel close and loving; what advice, suggestions, or support could the older wiser self give to help during these times (DeShazer, 1988)?

6. Have the couple make a list of things that each feels pleases their partner, or each feels the other would appreciate. Have the couple do at least one of these things for their partners between sessions. Have them do this privately, without discussion until this is shared the next session.

At some point during this Stage 1, stress increases. The stressor may stem from an increased environmental demand in "reality" (loss of a job, a family member become ill, geographical change, etc.), a perceived demand by one member of the couple, a biological (hormonal, nutritional) or dietary shift which lowers tolerance for stress (e.g., low blood sugar), a psychological demand (wife becomes pregnant, a child is flunking in school), a partner "distances" or "intrudes," or is perceived to do so, or an increase in social pressures. The increase in stress could be more internally generated (a disturbing thought, feeling, sensation, etc.) which one member becomes conscious of ("my wife is angry with me" based on his observation that she is quieter than usual; she is not home because she is having an affair; she is dressing nicely because she wants to attract other men; she shouldn't tell me what to do, after she makes a request of him, etc.).

As was discussed in the above research, and in accord with the cognitive approach to individual and marital therapy, we are concerned with a variety of cognitions in relationship problems. These, to summarize, refer to *perceptions, attributions, assumptions, values, unrealistic standards.* Also added to these are the images and thoughts and visual pictures that run through one's mind, and are associated with a variety of feelings (including physiological states of arousal). We will describe this process in detail in the next sections. Figures 1 and 2 outline the process which, whenever possible, is taught to the couple by the therapist and through bibliotherapy. Our hope is that clients will eventually become their own therapists, and this model can help in their work on themselves after they leave therapy.

STAGE 2: TENSION BUILDING (T2)

During the ongoing relationship one of the partners (Person 1 in the diagram) perceives (becomes aware of) something that troubles him/her (event A). This event could be an internal sensation or thought, an external event, such as a gesture, or behavior by the other, or even the omission of a happening where one was expected ("she didn't come home when she was supposed to"); the person then thinks about it (cognition). The event is given meaning; it is interpreted a certain way; this generates "self-talk," images, and associations that elaborate the meaning (Meichenbaum, 1977). The meaning (B) is a function of past experience (Parent, Adult and Child ego states, Berne, 1961), and the current (adult) assessment of the event, its context and its relationship to the person's self concept and concept of the other. If the meaning is dominated by "irrational" cognitions (Ellis, 1962), from the Parent and Child ego states (dysfunctional cognitions), the resultant feeling (C) is likely to be intense, negative, and painful (i.e., anger resulting from blaming the other; guilt from self blame; anxiety associated with future oriented catastrophizing; depression from thoughts of futility, helplessness and hopelessness, etc.). If the Adult ego state has the necessary "emotional muscle," the resultant thoughts and self talk will be rational, and the accompanying feelings appropriate (i.e., inconvenience, regret, concern, annoyance, hope, amusement, etc.).

An emotionally arousing event (A) is potentially anything a person becomes aware of which has psychological significance. This does not mean that a person is always fully conscious of the event and certain about its meaning. In fact, when working with clients, it takes hard work and persistence to "uncover" the activating event so that the client can understand that his behavior, and that of the other, did not occur without reason (and neither of them is "crazy"). The assumption is that there is always an

FIGURE 1. TARET SYSTEMS: Intra- and Interpersonal Flow Chart

WITNESS CONSCIOUSNESS
Non-judgmental Observer
(Provides feedback to Adult,
regarding what Adult, Parent
and Child is thinking, feeling
and doing)

Parent Ego State

SET 1   Conditioned Values and
attitudes; old tapes
affecting inner child;

Evaluations, judge-
ments and expectations
in moralistic terms
(i.e., irrational demands
and shoulds)

Adult Ego State
Accurate perceiver
(like video tape re-
corder); Reality
tester; computer;
Effective problem
solver; functions in
here and now; considers
short and long term
consequences

Child Ego State
a. Natural Child:
Innate emotional
and behavioral re-
sponse tendencies

b. Little Professor:
Innate intellect.
SET 2   potential; primitive
problem solving
efforts directed
to getting child
what it wants, when
and how it wants it;
Short term hedonism
and Intuitive source

c. Adapted Child:
Learned emotional,
Cognitive, and behavioral
response tendencies

EVENT A

1. Internal
e.g., sensations
thoughts and
fantasies

2. External
Interpersonal or
impersonal events

COGNITION

Perception and
Interpretations
of events; their
meaning; what
person says to
the self; all types
of cognitions–
Rational/irrational
functional/dysfunctional

AFFECT

Emotional arousal
Feelings experienced
in body and mind

RESPONSES

Behaviors learned as a function of past experience;
Behaviors reinforced through classical and/or
instrumental conditioning;
Responses emitted as a function of anticipated
Consequences ("payoffs", outcomes) be they
emotional, cognitive and behavioral effects in
the short or long run.

FIGURE 2. Integrative Holistic Stress Model

CONTEXT

SETS (Basic Assumptions)		AROUSING EVENTS	BELIEFS			
Cognitive Processes	Stressors	Cognitive	Mediators Processes	Resources	Outcomes
Expectation of Demands	Environmental Demands	Rational (Adult Ego)	Personality Factors: programmed patterns of thought, feelings and behaviors	Psychological Physical Social	Perceived and Actual Resources Exceed Demands
Expectation of efficacy	Psychological Physical Social Biological Demands	Irrational (Parent and Child Ego States)			Adaption Physiological Arousal is moderate and affect is appropriate
		Expectations, Assumptions, Appraisals, Attitudes, Images regarding perceived demands and efficacy	Social Conditions and Norms of Culture, Subculture, Family, etc.		Leads to effective problem solving
					Health is maintained

Maladaptive
Stress Reactions
Perceived
and
Actual demands
exceed
resources
Arousal is Intense and affect is negative;
Performance deficits or excesses regarding
problem solving;
Health is impaired

event, and our job is to (dis/un) cover it. This helps to reduce the mystical nature of the therapy process, and sets the stage for the client to work outside the therapy hour.

Some events "trigger" dysfunctional thoughts, feelings and behavior "sometimes." At other times the same behavior and events are negotiated without argument or violence. When this occurs, we ask clients to monitor the process for times when they are psychologically uncomfortable, under external or internal stress (due to illness, pressure, hormonal shifts, dietary induced reactions, environmental sensitivities, etc.), and this does not lead to destructive conflict. We are trying to discover the differences in the internal and external contexts that make a difference as to whether or not violence occurs.

Often several rational and irrational thoughts can co-exist, and cause a person to feel confused or undecided about what to conclude, feel or do. Under these conditions, the resultant response may be incongruent (i.e., the person's verbal and non-verbal reactions are inconsistent in that they convey contradictory information). The experienced "here and now" reactions (cognitively and emotionally) contribute to the responses, though they are limited by the constraints of the learned behavioral repertoire, and the person's cognitive ability to assess the potential consequences of his or her actions (i.e., what is the likelihood that they will produce the desired response in oneself or others, in terms of the emotional and behavioral consequences). Under the condition of intense emotional reactions, most clients produce self-defeating behaviors and emotions because their primary goal is to reduce discomfort or pain for a brief period, or as soon as possible (negative reinforcement), as opposed to generating long term gain (positive reinforcement). Addicts of all varieties, and especially angry, violent persons (Steinfeld, 1978), have low frustration tolerances, and irrational ideas that produce these negative affective and behavioral responses. Since the reduction of negative feelings is rewarding, impulsive and self defeating behavior is often reinforced, whereas positive, self-other enhancing behavior has either not been learned very well, or has a low probability of occurrence under stressful conditions (regressive tendencies). The main examples of this process are the different kinds of addicts we see every day (and this refers to most of us in one way or another, since, as many "addicts" have taught me, "you don't have to stick a needle in your arm to be a dope fiend"). The addictive coping pattern consists of responding to emotions like anger (mad), anxiety (scared), and depression (sad) in repeatedly self defeating ways, further generating these feelings in themselves and others (Steinfeld, 1978). Understanding interpersonal and intra-personal processes in this way creates a somewhat different view of "games" and "rackets" than has traditionally been formulated by Transactional Analysis. In T.A. literature (Berne, 1961; 1964; Erskine & Zalcman, 1979), clients are perceived to be motivated by "negative" intentions or unconscious forces. From a cognitive-behavioral, systems and spiritual perspective, people do the best they can at any moment of time, given their genetic and learning histories. This way of viewing patterns allows us to "positively connote" all behavior of clients (Selvini-Palazzoli, 1978), and to do so authentically without manipulation or unauthentic strategic or paradoxical methods. It also implies that if therapists get upset with clients, that it is their problem and they need to work on themselves before they can help their clients.

The response of Person 1 can be verbal or non-verbal (physical), congruent or incongruent (where the digital and analogic aspects of the message do not match in terms of their intended meaning). Even if Person 1 were to produce no overt response, Person 2 could perceive (interpret) a message via one of the sense modalities, intuitively or with full awareness, and the same internal (cognitive-emotional) process occurs. This internal process will culminate in another response which again will be perceived and interpreted by Person 1, and anyone else who is in the system, and involved in the communication process; this includes any and all members of the family, as well as the therapist, if the transactions are taking place in the office (Steinfeld, 1973). See the family diagram in Figure 3 for a schematic representation of this interpersonal process.

In violent relationships the "abusing" husband, or the "victimized" wife may trigger the sequence, and it is difficult to tease apart the opening gambit (the cue which initiates the series of moves leading to the eventual tissue damage). For example, the wife may begin to feel anxious about when the next violent episode will occur because her past experience tells her that violence is just around the corner. She may do something (e.g., "nag," become critical, spend money without checking with him, neglect her responsibilities) which might provoke her spouse. She may do this consciously (in order to gain some measure of control over a situation) or she may do this with dim awareness or without awareness of her motivations. In any case, she may be reacting to her anxiety over not knowing when her husband will "blow." She may also become anxious over her vulnerability due to her emotional closeness to her husband that is developing, her fear of being abandoned or hurt after being so close, her ambivalence about staying in the relationship which is violent, or any number of issues generated from her past or current relationship. She may also do "nothing" (which, from a communication and constructivist perspective, is impossible, since "nothing" can always be interpreted as "something").

The husband may start to feel anxious about feeling close, exposed, dependent, vulnerable. He may fear criticism (which arouses feelings of inadequacy already present in his self concept), being abandoned, or his own destructive impulses. He may react to what his wife has or hasn't done as a way of deflecting away from focusing on himself.

Both the husband and the wife, after many transactions in this and previous relationships, become sensitive to the subtle and not so subtle

FIGURE 3. TARET Schematic Family Interpersonal Diagram

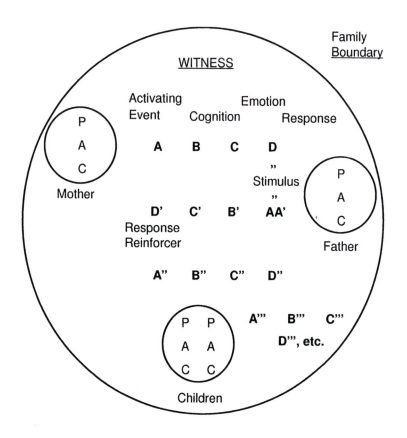

cues which may be interpreted irrationally (via schemas which have been conditioned as "filters" or "sets," leading to certain expectations and assumptions, causal attributions, which induce further anxiety and escalating conflict and ultimately violence. The escalation is due to the couple's lack of awareness of the cognitive-affective-behavioral sequence, their inability to see their own roles in provoking just the behavior they fear, their inability to communicate effectively, their lack of problem solving ability, and their unwillingness to accept themselves and each other in the interest of the relationship, as opposed to struggling to get what they want in the short run. All of these factors contribute to the final violent episode, and need to be teased apart during the therapeutic process.

Jacobson (1991) points out that the couple's rapid escalation of conflict, via their negative behavior, leads to a loss of their collaborative set, and that regression to a power struggle ensues, where a win-lose orientation comes into focus. This power struggle revolves around the issue of intimacy, or who controls how much intimacy will take place at any moment in time. Intimacy relates to the question of how close we will be, and how much one partner feels cared for. Caring is defined idiosyncratically. Clinically, we believe that when intimacy needs are not met, pain and anger emerge, and a struggle for control takes place. As discussed above, men and women fight differently, but women, most often, wind up battered, whereas men wind up isolated and alone.

Questions and Interventions Associated with the Tension Building State (T2)

The following questions are meant to help the couple increase their awareness of this tension building state so as to develop ways of managing their differences before the conflicts escalate into violence.

A. The Couple Relationship:

1. Just prior to the outburst of violence, describe what was happening.
2. You both were feeling good about each other (the hour, day, before); who first became aware of feeling uncomfortable, tense, upset, distant, etc.?
3. Describe what you first became aware of.
4. Think back and construct a picture so that we all can see it; what was happening just prior to the disagreement . . . Process this very closely. "Orange juice" the sequences so as to search for the antecedents (event A), and the dysfunctional cognitions surrounding the activating events.
5. Think back over your arguments (fights). Is there anything that triggers your upset feelings? Is there a general theme that can characterize your feelings? Have you ever felt this way in other situations (parents, teachers, etc.)?
6. How do you feel (in your body) when you are upset with your partner? Where in your body do you feel it? Describe the feelings, giving it some dimension (form, color, density, quality); explore its quality (stable, movement); see if the feeling changes or shifts as you focus your attention on it.
7. Is the feeling like anything you felt before? Explore the relationship between the past and the present. Rework the memories

associated with the current reactions, as in the work of David Grove, Richard Erskine's integrated T.A. approach, redecision therapy of Mary and Bob Goulding, or Zen therapy. Have the client stay with the feelings, focusing on them; does the client notice anything else besides the anger. Focusing on the bodily feeling may awaken a host of other feelings and memories which can be processed while the spouse listens and observes.

8. Can you think of anything you could have done or said that might produce a different response or outcome? How does it feel to do this right now (or in your imagination)?

B. For Family of Origin issues: (As you listen to clients describe their parents, or their interpretations of their parents' behavior, relate these projections to the clients and suggest they do the same).

1. How did your parents argue?
2. Who was most likely to start the fight?
3. What was it that he/she was responding to?
4. How did your (parent perpetrator) or (parent victim) stimulate the other parent to argue?
5. What was the purpose of your parent starting the fight?
6. Who do you think your children think start your fights? What would give them that idea?
7. How did you feel when your parents fought? How do you think your children feel? How do you know? Do you care?

C. Additional Interventions:

1. What can you do differently the next time that could prevent the escalation? What would make it worse?
2. Develop a set of options so that each partner can do something differently that would prevent the violence from occurring.
3. Stay with the different levels of work contracted for as will be described below.

THE CRISIS STAGE (T3)

The violent outburst is, as we have been describing, the result of many past and present factors that mediate between the precipitating stressor and the eventual destructive behavior. These factors can be separated into two categories: the first is "personality" (programmed patterns of perception, thought, feeling and action tendencies in response to stress). These patterns are conceived to be based on innate predispositions as well as past learning or conditioning histories.

The second category has to do with the social conditions that exist surrounding the violence (that is, the context in which the stressors are occurring, who is doing what to whom, where, what is contaminating and contributing to the stress, etc. If a person's resources, physical, psychological, social, exceed the perceived demand, the response will be adaptive. The problem will be solved, no violence will occur, and the couple will move on with a sense of competency that they can work out their difficulties and resolve the conflicts in ways that could bring them even closer together. When the perceived demand exceeds the perceived resources, we have a maladaptive stress reaction which manifests itself in a high state of physiological arousal, negative affect, and a performance deficit, that is, violence; long term problem solving has failed, health is impaired, the relationship continues to be in jeopardy, the couple is hurting emotionally and the woman is likely to also be hurting physically. And if recent research on the mind-body relationship holds, anger and hostility are cardiovascular risk factors for the man as well.

There are different levels of violence from verbal haranguing, demeaning language, coercion, threats and intimidation, through pushing and shoving, restraining, to physical assault with and without a weapon. How these behaviors are interpreted is a function of the perpetrators and victim's perception and attitudes toward violence. If the receiver of the response perceives it as abuse, it is (at least psychologically, although it may not have passed the threshold of illegal behavior). Nevertheless, the couple is in difficulty and the interactional pattern needs to change. If a person does not feel that her partner's behavior is abusive, it may still be, according to the law. Thus, in Connecticut, if the police are called by anyone, and if they see that a person has been physically hurt, an arrest is made, regardless of whether either partner claims that abuse has occurred. This approach has proponents and opponents, but, on the national level, arrests by police who have been called into domestic disputes are correlated with a reduction of domestic violence in those states that have this law.

After the escalation of conflict, and the violent outburst, there is the immediate reinforcement in that the anxiety has been momentarily reduced, and there is gratification of the aggressive impulse. This is why abusive spouses can be characterized as addicts (Steinfeld, 1978) who sacrifice long term pain for short term gain. However, the long term consequences still occur and must eventually be dealt with by both parties.

Questions Regarding "Personality" Factors and Social Conditions Surrounding Violence

A. Personality:

1. How have your dealt with the stressors related to anger in the past?
2. How come when you're angry at X (e.g., your boss, your friend, your mother, etc.) you don't yell or strike out, but you do this with your wife? These type of questions are geared toward making the perpetrator aware that he, in fact, can control the way he expresses his anger, and even experience it. He is helped to become aware of the antecedents and consequences of violence, and how these affect his decision to behave in certain ways in different contexts.
3. How long have you lashed out at people close to you (at X, your partner, other women, etc.). Who did what when you did so (search for reinforcing consequences that helped teach the perpetrator that it was acceptable to use force and violence to get what he wanted; was abuse modeled in his family of origin; was it justified, etc.)?
4. What did you feel just before you felt the anger (to help men learn that other feelings precede or accompany the anger, e.g., guilt, fear, helplessness, etc.).
5. Have you ever expressed feelings of pain (fear, sadness, helplessness, guilt, shame) to your wife? What effect do you think it would have it you did? What would it be like for you to do this?
6. Imagine yourself expressing these "softer" feelings to her. What does she say or do in response to you. How do you feel when you do this? How do you feel about yourself? Not only do men have problems expressing these softer feelings, but women may "punish" men for doing so, calling them "wimps" or in some way implying that they are unmanly, and reinforcing the man's perception that he is weak if he does express these feelings.

B. Family of Origin issues:

1. How did your parents negotiate or settle their differences?
2. Did your parents express other feelings toward each other? When?
3. In what ways are you similar/different from your mother/father/ other care taker?

4. Were you ever abused or a witness to it in your family? What was it like. What did you do or want to do? What happened during the fight between your parents?

C. Present Factors:

1. When you want something from your wife/husband, how do you communicate this (are they asking/demanding to get what they want)? What is your partner's response to how you ask/demand what you want?
2. What, who, is around when you fight? Who isn't? Where do you fight (place); what is the time of day or night? Look for any condition that is part of the pattern so as to develop leads to help shift the context of their future arguments.
3. Pay attention to what you feel, think and do when you overcome your urge to lash out.

CONTRITE STAGE (T4)

In violent relationships, the perpetrator, seeing what he has done, may act remorseful, and ask for forgiveness from the victim. No matter how severely or how frequently she has been battered, experience shows that she is likely to forgive him, or at least act as if she does. Her motivations for doing this may be complicated, that is, because she still "loves" him (whatever that means; this needs to be explored in therapy), for economic reasons, or for social or other psychological reasons, including the children. Even if she calls the police (or someone else does), if they come (and they tend to do so more now than in years gone by, at least in Connecticut), if charges are filed (even though she may not want them to be), if she gets a restraining order for several months (which she may or may not employ), or even if she goes to a shelter for a period of time (with her children, if there are any), the evidence indicates that she is likely to return home, or that the perpetrator is allowed to do so, most of the time (80-90%). The escalating conflict, abuse and separation has generated so much anxiety relating to the loss of one another, that each spouse will do what he/she thinks he/she has to do to restore the equilibrium (and calmness, at least for a little time) and thereby avoid further anxiety associated with ending the relationship.

If the batterer is not actually remorseful, but feels that he has established his "rightful" control through violence, or threats of it, his female partner will usually accept him back so that calmness is again restored. Frequently, intense intimacy-provoking behavior follows the reconciliation, in the form of increased sexual activity, going out for recreational activities, and helpfulness around the house and with the kids, all of which reinforce the couple's "loving" relationship, not to mention the delusion that the violence will not happen again.

Her willingness to act as though she forgives him, though she clearly never forgets his actions, and is ever vigilant for their return (at least after the first few cycles; before this she may have believed that his violence was an isolated event), her actions reinforce his violent behavior, and stamps in her victimization. This way of acting also reinforces her help-lessness, and robs her of her power to change the situation. Even her attempts to get help from the police and from mental health professionals may have failed, and even if she and her partner were to enter treatment, the evidence is that therapists do not like to focus on his violence, or to offer crisis intervention (e.g., shelter recommendations) when she is in danger of being battered again. Contracts are additional attempts to protect her (Steinfeld, 1989).

The only way out for the victim is for her to engage in new behavior that makes it clear that she will no longer accept his definition of the relationship, and his use of force to control her. If she can summon her internal resources related to her autonomy, and if she has the emotional and legal support system to validate her, and her right to stand up and assert her right not to be coerced or forced to do what she does not want to do (in T.A. therapy, this offers her the Permission and Protection she needs), she may be able to negotiate a new role for herself and change the nature of the relationship (Potency). Under these conditions, calmness may be restored, but in a new way. If he rejects her new behavior, the crisis will continue, so that the law may eventually be called in to settle matters, to protect her from further threats and violence, although, all too frequent-ly, even the police cannot stop a enraged husband or lover intent on maintaining the status quo and his right to control the nature of the rela-tionship with his female partner. But if he is incarcerated for his behavior, then society has protected the victim in ways she could not do for herself (although he may be so enraged and vindictive that he may taunt and want to hurt her after being released from prison, so that a victim may never really feel safe). Sometimes, although rarely, the abuser himself seeks help for the violent behavior that he knows is destructive to himself, his wife and the children. Needless to say, the prognosis for change is best in these cases, although the work to actually help the man change is never easy.

If the calmness can be restored by any of the above mechanisms, it will continue until levels of intimacy develop to the point that anxiety is again generated by the closeness, the "catastrophic expectations" that closeness arouses, or by other kinds of stress that the man is unable to manage in a healthy and functional way. Again, responses to the stress may stimulate behaviors that start the cycle again, so that the same pattern repeats itself over and over (perhaps, "until death do us part").

Questions Exploring the Contrite Stage (T4)

A. Current Relationship

1. Why did you return to the relationship? What did you hope would happen if you returned?
2. What does happen after the abuse?
3. How do you make up?
4. Do you believe him when he says he's sorry? Do you believe yourself when you say you believe him or accept him back?
5. Do you believe yourself when you apologize (him)?
6. How frequently will this have to happen before you stop (him); stop believing he's really sorry (her)?
7. How will you know that he's working on himself to stop hurting you?
8. What will you do to prevent further abuse? Provoke further abuse?
9. Have you both agreed on what you both will do if further abuse happens (contract)?
10. If you feel that you provoke your partner, what is it you are trying to accomplish? How is it useful?

B. Family of Origin

1. When your parents argued, with or without violence, how did they make up?
2. How did you make up with your parent, siblings, when you fought with them?
3. Who is responsible for your anger and your violence? Who is responsible for your actions with your husband?

BEHAVIORAL EFFECTS

In the current cognitive-behavioral-systems model, a behavioral response may serve a number of functions. The clinical approach has the underlying assumptions that there is circular causality involved in the interpersonal process, and that we can intervene at any point in the process to alter the outcome. From a cognitive-communications framework (constructivist meta-theory) (Mahoney, 1990) a behavior is clearly a response to an antecedent internal or external stimulus. It may act as a reinforcer of prior responses, and it may even function as a stimulus to oneself or others (another antecedent). Behavior, as learning theorists have clearly demonstrated, is often a function of its consequences, even if these consequences are anticipated in thought, as most cognitively oriented therapists would agree. Behavior is also functional, that is, it is purposive and goal directed, as cognitive learning theorists, from Tolman on (1935), would accept. One purpose is to produce an effect on the environment (or the people in it). One may or may not be aware of the effects of one's behavior, especially the long term effects. From an observer's point of view, it is the meaning of the response (its cognitive-emotional effect on the receiver) which determines the subsequent response. What is intended regarding the meaning of the sent message may have nothing to do with the meaning the receiver attributes to the message. "I love you, that's why I'm so jealous (and want to control your every move)" may be the message sent, but this kind of love is very confusing to the recipient who has violated the sender's expectation and has been battered as a result. If love equals control equals physical force and abuse, these confusing messages can drive someone crazy (and I have heard many children and women say this about their abusive fathers and husbands).

The "meaning of the message is in the response to it" (a position consistent with constructivist philosophy, Feffer, 1988). People are often not consciously aware of the effects of their behavior on others (denial), or are not willing to think or say what they know to be the effects (lying), or do not know or state what effects they want to have. Very few, if any, abusers will say "I want to control my wife." Rather, they say things like, "she should do X; if she loved me she would do X; she's my wife and has to X," etc. It is useful to ask questions dealing with intention or purpose, e.g., what did you want to accomplish; what effect did you want to have; what was the purpose of what you did; what was the effect, etc.

From a psychodynamic perspective, we can ask "why" people abuse one another, and why victims stay (beyond the frequently discussed factors like economic and emotional dependency). Victims (survivors) frequently blame themselves for the violence their spouses heap on them, a belief that the batterer is quick to support. It takes a great deal of work and skill to convince women that they are not responsible for their partners' violent behavior, and, as stated, most do not leave. If they believe they are not responsible, and stay for other reasons, these still need to be investigated. An "old" dynamic explanation of victim abuse blamed her by calling her masochistic, and blaming the victim is still a frequent phenomenon in our culture. Freud's "repetition compulsion" fueled the masochistic explanation. But a more optimistic framing of the motivations of victims and perpetrators is that each has been wounded by persons in their past, and has selected one another with characteristics similar to those in the past who have hurt them so as to, hopefully, change the outcome in the present. Unfortunately, without help to tease apart past from present, persons are destined to repeat the earlier negative experiences, reinforcing their negative self appraisals. No research exists to justify these dynamic formulations of dysfunctional abusive patterns, but if they are offered, and individuals and couples are willing to use them to change, they could prove useful, since they eliminate blame, while holding each responsible for the change. After all, the concept of "blameless responsibility" is consistent with many psychological and spiritual approaches to helping and healing.

In Eastern spiritual thought, short and long term behavioral effects are referred to as karma. From a cognitive-constructivist perspective, to be in control of one's life is to be aware (conscious) of the entire process:

a. The internal and external antecedents and consequences of one's reactions (seeing them arising and disappearing),
b. being able to control one's behavior to produce the most desirable effects.

This awareness enables one to choose the most appropriate responses on the basis of the "probable" long and short term effects on oneself and others, as they occur over time. This is the essence of personal freedom, limited as it may be. Developing one's "center," by improving one's ability to move toward, and make contact with one's "witness" (the nonjudgmental, self accepting, part of the self) can foster awareness, compassion, and self control. Being centered in one's witness allows for emotional spontaneity, creativity, and rational (functional) decision making, which, in turn, improves one's sense of balance (continuity and change). Not only do a person's responses (internal and external) affect others, but each person "witnesses" his or her own thoughts, feelings, and behavior, thereby receiving feedback in a never ending circular process.

ADDITIONAL GUIDELINES IN WORKING WITH VIOLENT COUPLES

The writer, in agreement with Avis (1992), believes that the following guidelines are helpful when working with individuals and couples:

1. Abusive men must be seen as responsible for their actions and be held accountable for it no matter what the mitigating circumstances or so-called provocative behavior of their partners. Therapists must not collude with the abuser's denial, minimization, avoidance of responsibility and projections, or by "taking his partner's inventory" to account for his behavior.
2. The main purpose of therapy is the cessation of abuse. Other goals are important but secondary (self esteem issues, better communication and problem solving, etc.) Stopping violence must be the contract.
3. Therapists must be able to work within the larger social system, in conjunction and cooperation with police, the courts, battered women's services, and other social service agencies.

The model of therapy presented here takes a feminist perspective into account. However, my experience tells me that matters are not so simple, nor are they black or white regarding how to work with perpetrators and couples. We can try to understand and be empathic with the perpetrator's experience, while we still hold him fully accountable for his behavior. We can work to help him change his thoughts and actions, yet we can and have to collaborate with the court system and the police to use legal sanctions to mandate treatment for most perpetrators who may deny their need for it. In fact, I am not so certain that treatment options are *always* useful. I am not aware of the research which confirms that our therapy approaches reduce violence, even though our experience indicates that it does help. We clinicians have not been immune to fooling ourselves into believing that our treatments are effective in reducing suffering, only to discover that there is no research to support our assumptions. We might discover that prison does a more effective job in reducing partner violence, at least with some men.

The writer supports the view that we can be both therapists and social control agents, but I also know that much research is needed to determine what types of offenders, with what developmental, personality, and behavioral characteristics, in what contexts, with what types of women, under what stressful conditions, are most amenable to what kinds of therapy, and which offender, and the persons he has harmed, are best served by incarceration.

In developing treatment guidelines, the writer's experience corresponds to that of Kaufman (1992), and he concurs with many (but clearly not all) of his suggestions of how to support the less powerful victim of abuse, the woman, while helping the man to change.

1. Kaufman suggests that a woman therapist be part of the treatment, and that "ideally, the woman therapist will have been through volunteer training at a battered women's shelter."

Comment: Although it may be useful to have a woman present during couple work, the writer, as most therapists, works alone most of the time. The level of danger is assessed from what the individuals say, alone and together, how they say it, their past history of violence, understanding that most batterers minimize, deny, or lie about the frequency, intensity, duration and type of violence they have committed. The violence tactics scale is also used to assess past behavior and potential for future risk. The writer does not consider it vital to have a woman therapist in the room. When there has been a female co-therapist, what was important was her frame of reference, experience as a therapist, level of consciousness, and what unfinished business she might still be working through regarding gender, power, control, and violence issues, including her own.

2. Kaufman suggests that we ask the following:

   a. What happens when you argue?
   b. Has he ever hit or shoved you?
   c. Are you afraid of what he might do if you didn't back down?

In deciding on the level of the man's controlling behavior, ask yourself, "What if he'd done it to you."

Comment: These are useful questions. The man can also be asked: "How would he feel if what he had done to his partner, someone has done to him?" This opens many therapeutic doors.

3. If the therapist "sniffs" violence, separate the couple, with a man seeing the man, and a woman seeing the woman. The woman can work on a safety plan, what she can do to maximize her safety.

Comment: The writer prefers to see each partner alone, whether or not violence is related to the presenting problem. Experience indicates that individuals are more open and honest about what is bothering them when seen alone. If violence potential exists, a safety plan is always developed, and a non-violent contract is established (Steinfeld, 1989).

4. Kaufman suggests that we refer the woman to the nearest battered woman's shelter. One can be located by calling 1-800-333-SAFE, the National Domestic Violence hotline (for the hearing impaired,

call 1-800-873-6363). He reports that shelters have legal advocacy and woman support groups. "There she'll hear women tell stories, she won't feel isolated and crazy anymore. The staff won't tell her what to do; they work on the principle of helping to empower her to make her own decisions. Even if she doesn't go now, she'll have the number for the next time."

Comment: The writer is sorry to say that not all battered women's groups operate with such therapeutic skill. The writer has heard many stories from women who have been to these groups, in and out of shelters, in which counselors have encouraged them to leave their partners, and have told them that batterers cannot change, and what they "should do" in many ways. The writer is not saying that all of us are so therapeutically detached that we have not actively or subtly suggested to clients our preferences for what we feel they "should do," but to imply that all staff at all shelters act non-judgementally and are unbiased is, from the writer's experience, naive.

5. If the woman gives you the okay, Kaufman suggests that the therapist tell the abuser why you won't do couples therapy–you don't believe it will be safe for his partner, and you won't go along to keep him from feeling upset, controlled or uncomfortable. Tell him that what he has done is a crime, that this is a criminal matter, not a therapeutic issue (even though they undoubtedly have individual and couple problems). Tell him you believe it is his job to stop endangering her, to do what is necessary for her to feel safe, though she may never feel safe around him again.

Comment: These are excellent suggestions, and the writer supports them. A therapist can do all this, including taking an active stance of suggesting to a woman what you feel is in her best interest, and still do couples therapy. What is required is directness and honesty about what you will or will not do, and this is where a non-violence contract, spelling out everyone's expectations and responsibilities, is important to consider.

6. Finally, Kaufman suggests getting supervision by battered women's advocates. "Build in listening to women in contexts where they are free and empowered to speak the truth. Read feminist literature and battered women's books. There we can't intimidate or interrupt, or force a book to placate us" (p. 241).

Comment: Again, the writer has little quarrel with Kaufman's suggestions, except "getting supervision from battered women's advocates." The writer has presented his ideas to battered women's agencies, and rape crisis counselors, and would not refer women to many of these persons because of the clinical inexperience, their lack of training in psychological and systems theory and practice, their tendency to project their own experiences onto all women, and not see the unique person and her circumstances, her developmental history, and her values and goals for herself and her family. I do not want to generalize from my experiences to all staff at all agencies. I am certain that many are well trained, and systems oriented. But neither do I assume that because a staff person has had some training and has been the victim of battering that automatically makes her an effective therapist with all battered women. Also, the writer has found that these ideas when presented to battered women's counselors are more readily accepted if the same messages are delivered by female colleagues who share a similar perspective.

SOME WORDS REGARDING FAMILY SYSTEMS THERAPY WITH VIOLENT COUPLES

Systemic, interactional neutrality is therapeutic for many issues and interpersonal problems, but not in cases of family violence. Therapeutic neutrality in these cases are acts of omission (thereby subtly reinforcing the status quo) and, as a result, contributes to the maintenance of the problem. Many battered women and men services have clear definitions of power, control, and violence, and facilitate the change process by making the hidden and denied more visible, and experientially real. Some family therapists go even further by working in ways that are both respectful to men, and curious about the relationship, while reframing processes in ways that go beyond intrapsychic and interpersonal explanations by labeling the woman's exploitation and the man's control and violence (Goldner, Penn, Scheinberg & Walker, 1990). The writer finds this approach consistent with his. More specifically, a therapist can search for the positive intent of the perpetrator's actions, even his violence, and still focus on the negative and destructive outcomes, while holding the perpetrator responsible and accountable for these acts. When Bograd (1992) asks, "What would it mean for us to acknowledge openly that we are simultaneously doing therapy and are exerting social control," the answer is, "It would mean that we are being honest," and the writer sees no problem or inconsistency in doing just this.

The current clinical model can "interweave psychological, interpersonal, political and legal dimensions," as Bograd suggests (p. 250), as the optimal stance for therapists. Although we can be advocates for women, while still maintaining a therapeutic position in relation to the couple, the feminist literature often views the man as operating in isolation, and not part of a complicated dynamic relationship, influenced not only by the current partners, but by all the other people who are still living in the heads of the couple.

Again, it is clear that the man is responsible for his abusive behavior, no matter what the internal or external, intended or unintended, provocation has been to which he responded. But women, in much of the feminist literature the writer has read, and the talks to which he has listened, seem to play no other role than being the victim or survivor of the violence. To state that a woman has a role in creating and maintaining relationship problems is not to deny that she has been violated by the abuse of her partner, that he is responsible for the effects of his destructive behavior, and that he needs to face the consequences of his actions (e.g., the legal and relationships consequences, not to mention the effects on himself).

FUTURE CONSIDERATIONS

It seems that the next area of development of clinical approaches to family violence will focus on specific interventions by which to join with specific types of batterers and couples. Typologies are starting to emerge for perpetrators of child abuse (Finklhor's recent study mentioned in Lear, 1992), and experience tells us that men batter for different reasons, and under different conditions. Knowing this helps us develop more specific interventions, thereby reducing treatment time (increased efficiency) and increasing effectiveness, and making treatment, using these criteria, more ethical. We know that most batterers are resistant to focus on themselves as responsible for their abusive behavior, and needing change, preferring to blame their partners for their actions. As we clinicians continue to elicit information which sheds light on their belief systems, we can then develop intervention strategies which can facilitate change at the level of treatment contracted for. DeShazer is using his brief treatment model to develop computer simulated interventions for family treatment in general. Brief treatment approaches have been used with adolescent substance abusers, and Eve Lipchick is employing DeShazer's model with violent couples. How effective these approaches are still needs to be evaluated, as do other forms of treatment for batterers and their partners. In the future, we may be able to use this approach for specific types of batterers, working individually or in groups, and with violent couples and families. Although the main goal of treatment is the elimination of violence, we need to keep in mind that the violence comes out of and has created pain for the entire family, and each member requires healing in their own special way. While we may want treatment to be as brief and effective as possible, thereby making it ethical (Haley, 1975), it needs to take as much time as needed for the entire family to heal from the wounds the violence has inflicted. In this way not only will we break the cycle of violence within the couple, but, hopefully, we break the generational transmission process of destructive family behavior.

REFERENCES

Bandler, R., & Grinder, J. (1982). *Neurolinguistic Programming and Transformation of Meaning.* Real People Press, Moab, Utah.

Baucom, D. H. (1995). Four F.A.C.T.s of marriage: Forgiveness, Acceptance, Commitment, and Trust. *Symposium 40,* American association of Behavior therapy, New York.

Beck, A. (1976). *Cognitive Therapy and the Emotional Disorders.* International Universities Press, New York.

Berne, E. (1961). *Transactional Analysis in Psychotherapy.* Grove Press, New York.

Berne, E. (1964). *Games People Play: The Psychology of Human Relationships.* New York: Grove Press.

Bograd, M. (1984). Family systems approaches to wife battering: A feminist critique. *American Journal of Orthopsychiatry, 54,* 558-568.

Campbell, J.C. (1990). Battered woman syndrome: A critical review. *Violence: Update, December,* 1, 4, 10-11.

Dell, P. (1989). Violence and the systemic view: The problem of power. *Family Process, 28,* 1-14.

Deschner, J.P.(1984). *The Hitting Habit.* The Free Press, New York.

DeShazer, S. (1982). *Patterns of Brief Family Therapy: An Ecosystemic Approach.* New York: Guilford.

Douglas, M.A. (1987). The battered woman syndrome. In D. Sonkin (Ed.), *Domestic Violence on Trial.* New York: Springer.

Dutton, D.G. (1988). *The Domestic assault of Women.* Newton, MA: Allyn and Bacon.

Dutton, D. G. (1995). Intimate violence. *Clinical Psychology, 2,* 3, 207-225.

Ellis, A. (1962). *Reason and emotion in psychotherapy.* Citadel Press, Secaucus, N.J.

Erskine, R., & Zalcman, M. (1979). The racket system: a model for racket analysis. *Transactional Analysis Journal, 9,* 1, 51-59.

Farrington, K. (1986). The application of stress theory to family violence: Principles, problems and prospects. *Journal of Family Violence, 1,* 131-147.

Feffer, M. (1988). *Radical Constructionism.* New York: New York University Press.

Finklehor, D., & Williams, L.M. (1992). Characteristics of incest offenders. In Incest: A Chilling Report, *Lears,* February, 60-61.

Goldner, V., Penn, P., Scheinberg, M., & Walker, G. (1990). Love and violence: Gender paradoxes in volatile attachments. *Family process, 29 (No. 4)*, 343-363.

Gondolph, E.W. (1988). *Battered Women as Survivors.* D.C. Heath: Lexington Books.

Goulding, R., & Goulding, M. (1979). *Changing lives through redecision therapy.* New York: Bruner/Mazel.

Haley, J. (1976). *Problem Solving Therapy.* Jossey Bass, San Francisco.

Harris, T. (1973). *I'm Okay, You're Okay.* New York: Avon.

Jacobson, N.S. (1989). The politics of intimacy. *The Behavior Therapist, 12*, 29-32.

Jacobson, N. (1991). Cognitive interventions in couples and families. *Helping people change.* (2 tapes). Portoloa Valley, CA: IAHB.

Kaufman, G. (1992) The mysterious disappearance of battered women in family therapists' offices: Male privilege colluding with male violence. *Journal of Marriage & Family Therapy, 18*, 3, 233-244.

Kurz, D., & Stark, E. (1988). Not-so-benign neglect: The medical response to battering. In K. Yllo & M. Bograd (Eds.), *Feminist Perspectives on Wife Abuse.* Newbury Park, CA: Sage.

Mahoney, M. (1974). *Cognition and Behavior Modification.* Cambridge, MA: Ballinger.

Meichenbaum, D. (1977). *Cognitive Behavior Modification.* Plenum, New York.

Morrison, R.L., Van Hasselt, V.B., & Bellack, A.S. (1987). Assessment of assertion and problem solving skills in wife abusers and their spouses. *Journal of Family Violence, 2*, 227-238.

Murphy, C.M., & Meyer, S.L. (1991). Gender, power, and violence in marriage. *The behavior therapist, 14 (4)*, 95-100.

Novaco, R. (1979). The cognitive regulation of anger and stress. In Kendall, P.C., & Hollon, S.D. (Eds.), *Cognitive Behavior Interventions: Theory, Research and Procedures,* Academic Press, New York.

O'hanlon, B., & Wilk, J. (1987). *Shifting Contexts.* New York: Guilford.

O'Leary, K.D., Cascardi, M. (1994). Physical aggression in marriage: a developmental analysis. In *The developmental course of marital dysfunction* T.N. Bradbury (Ed.), Cambridge University Press.

Ram Dass. (1976). *Grist for the Mill.* Anchor Books, Santa Cruz, CA.

Schwartz, M.D. (1987). Gender and injury in spousal assault. *Sociological Focus, 20*, 61-74.

Seligman, M. (1975). *Helplessness: On Depression, Development and Death.* San Francisco: Freeman.

Seligman, M., & Maier, S.F. (1976). Learned helplessness: Theory and evidence. *Journal of Experimental Psychology: General, 105*, 3-46.

Selvini-Palazzoli, M., Cecchin, G., Prata, G., & Boscolo, L. (1978). *Paradox and Counterparadox: A New Model in the Therapy of the Family in Schizophrenic Transaction.* New York: Aronson.

Steinfeld, G.J. (1973). Experiential behavior therapy with families: A systems approach. *Journal of Clinical Child Psychology, 2,* 34-37.

Steinfeld, G.J. (1975). A theoretical basis for rational emotive psychotherapy. *Institute for Rational Therapy,* New York.

Steinfeld, G.J. (1978a). Decentering and family process: A marriage of cognitive therapies. *Journal of Marriage & Family Counseling, 4,* 61-70.

Steinfeld, G.J. (1978b). Dope fiend irrationality: It takes one to know one. *Psychotherapy: Theory, Research, Practice, 15,* 193-200.

Steinfeld, G.J. (1980). *TARET SYSTEMS: An Integrative Approach to Marriage and Family Therapy.* Pilgrimage Press, Jonesboro, TN.

Steinfeld, G.J. (1981). Establishing treatment contracts in family therapy. In Gurman, A.S. (ed.), *Questions and Answers in the Practice of Family Therapy,* Guilford, New York.

Steinfeld, G.J. (1989). Spouse abuse: An integrative-interactional model. *Journal of Family Violence, 4,* 1-23.

Steinfeld, G.J. (1995). Shifting perspective: An integrative approach to personal and interpersonal psychotherapy, *in process.*

Vanderbilt, H. (1992). Incest: A chilling report. *Lears, February,* 50-77.

Walker, L. (1979). *The Battered Woman.* Harper & Row, New York.

Walker, L. (1984). *The Battered Woman Syndrome.* New York: Springer.

Watzlawick, P, Weakland, J., & Fisch, R. (1974). *Change: Principles of Problem Formation and Problem Resolution.* Norton, New York.

Zuckerman, C., & Rock, I. (1957). A reappraisal of the roles of past experience and innate organizing principles in visual perception. *Psychological Bulletin, 54,* 269-296.

A Cross-Cultural Perspective
on Couple Differences

Margaret A. Waller
Michael D. Spiegler

SUMMARY. This paper challenges the idea that differences between partners in couple relationships are inherently problematic. A
"cross-cultural" perspective on differences in couples that considers
partners' *reactions* to difference as the problem is presented. Couples therapy from a cross-cultural perspective begins with a detailed
assessment of perceived differences, reactions to differences, the
context in which the differences have developed, and the purposes
they serve. Therapeutic tasks involve managing maladaptive reactions to differences, learning to accept differences, and co-designing
a common couple culture. *[Article copies available for a fee from The
Haworth Document Delivery Service: 1-800-342-9678. E-mail address:
getinfo@haworth.com]*

Differences between partners in a couples relationship are inevitable.
Yet, both clients and therapists frequently view *difference* as a problem to
be "fixed." We believe that this view is inherently flawed. A "cross-cultural" perspective on differences in couples considers partner's *reactions*

Margaret A. Waller, PhD, is Assistant Professor, School of Social Work,
Rhode Island College, Providence, RI 02908.

Michael D. Spiegler, PhD, is Professor, Department of Psychology, Providence College, Providence, RI 02918.

Send correspondence to Dr. Waller at: 5 Tanglewood Road, N. Smithfield, RI
02896.

[Haworth co-indexing entry note]: "A Cross-Cultural Perspective on Couple Differences." Waller,
Margaret A., and Michael D. Spiegler. Co-published simultaneously in *Journal of Couples Therapy*
(The Haworth Press, Inc.) Vol. 7, No. 1, 1997, pp. 83-98; and: *When One Partner Is Willing and the
Other Is Not* (ed: Barbara Jo Brothers) The Haworth Press, Inc., 1997, pp. 83-98. Single or multiple
copies of this article are available for a fee from The Haworth Document Delivery Service [1-800-342-9678,
9:00 a.m. - 5:00 p.m. (EST). E-mail address: getinfo@haworth.com].

83

to difference as the problem. Accordingly, it often is more useful for couples to begin by learning to accept differences rather than attempting to resolve or eliminate them. Once there is acceptance, it is possible for partners to co-design a common culture that preserves the essential elements of each partner's personal culture.

Culture has been defined as the beliefs, assumptions, values, understandings, images, and symbols that guide a group's thinking and behaving (Hurvitz & Straus, 1991). Broadly interpreted, culture applies to individuals as well as to groups. We believe it is useful to think of each individual as having a *personal culture,* which is the product of a combination of ethnic, socioeconomic, familial, life-experience, and within-person factors. Thus, even individuals who come from the same (group) culture will have different personal cultures. Indeed, individuals' personal cultures, like their personalities, are unique (cf. Liebert & Spiegler, 1994). In this paper we will use the term *cross-cultural* to refer to the mix of two *personal* cultures.

A couple, then, always is composed of two individuals with different personal cultures. Differences in sex, age, biological rhythm, education, occupation, beliefs, values, norms, meaning systems, expectations, behavior patterns, pacing, coping strategies, and communication style are commonplace. Furthermore, each partner enters a relationship with a full set of values and expectations about couple and family organization. For instance, each partner has preconceived ideas about optimal boundaries, including such variables as: frequency of contact; extent of involvement in one anothers' lives; interdependence versus autonomy; the balance of individual versus couple welfare; and the inclusion of others in the relationship (Shaver, Hazan, & Bradshaw, 1988). Individuals' ideas about the nature of an ideal relationship often are tacit, which in no way diminishes their powerful influence on the relationship (Bagarozzi & Anderson, 1989).

Each person also brings to a couple relationship a personal code of conduct that defines the "right" way of doing things. It does not take long for each partner to realize that the other is doing some things the "wrong" way. The unfamiliar challenges the sanctity of the known. Intimacy with a different other arouses fear that what is essential to oneself may be changed or lost (Axelson, 1993). For example, one couple had a disastrous first Christmas together because while one partner was out shopping, the other, with the best intentions of sharing the work, erected and decorated the Christmas tree. Upon returning, the second partner was greatly distressed because, in that partner's family of origin, it was an unspoken rule that putting up and decorating the tree was a collaborative family affair.

Couples enter therapy with both similarities and differences. Yet, it is differences that immediately surface—generally in the form of complaints—and typically remain the focus of therapy. Frequently, differences are what the couple has come to therapy to "fix." The familiar refrain couples therapists hear is: "Why can't my partner be more like me?" (Braverman, 1995)—which is reminiscent of Henry Higgin's equally naive question (in *My Fair Lady*), "Why can't a woman be more like a man?"

The predominant view, among clients and therapists alike, is that difference is an impediment to relationships and the degree of difficulty experienced is proportional to the degree of difference (Reiss, 1976). When difference is viewed as a liability, it is pathologized and mistakenly made a problem to be solved rather than an inevitable feature of couple relationships. This perspective is reflected in the quantity of therapeutic air time devoted to differences as problems. Even the language of dissolution of relationships speaks of "irreconcilable differences."

An opposing minority view suggests that difference is a valuable resource for couples (Winch, 1955). It is based on the idea that an integration of two complementary ways of living may provide a richer whole than a more homogeneous partnership (as might be the case if one partner were work-oriented and the other were relationship-oriented). It also has been suggested that interpersonal difference can provide the opportunity for increased personal development for both partners (Axelson, 1993). However, while it is true that differences may lead to a more creative approach to living, couples therapists who subscribe indiscriminantly to this view may idealize differences and consequently may fail to acknowledge and deal with distress related to differences.

We suggest that differences in themselves are neither liabilities nor assets in couple relationships—a position that is consistent with the stance taken by clinicians who work with diverse populations (e.g., Atkinson & Hackett, 1995; Atkinson, Morten, & Sue, 1989; Falicov & Brudner-White, 1986; Pinderhughes, 1989). Rather, the partners' perceptions of their differences have the potential to undermine or enhance a relationship. In fact, the same behaviors may be perceived differently at various times, as when partners are repelled by the very behaviors that they initially found appealing. For example, the showering of attention and desire to be together that was viewed as flattering during courtship may later be seen as suffocating.

A couple's inability to deal effectively with differences is not only a source of friction but, more significantly, it interferes with mutually satisfying intimacy. An intimate relationship requires a sense of freedom to be one's uncensored self in the presence of the loved one. Because intimacy involves extensive self-disclosure, intimate partners cannot conceal essential parts of themselves without jeopardizing the relationship.

When a couple's distress is seen as arising from the partners' *difficulty in dealing with* inevitable differences, therapy focuses on helping the couple acknowledge, accept, and work with differences. An overriding goal of cross-cultural couples therapy is for partners to develop an adaptive and flexible view of differences in each other's personal cultures. This makes it possible for the couple to maintain essential individual beliefs and practices, negotiate areas of conflict, and co-design an idiosyncratic cultural code that integrates both cultural streams (Falicov & Brudner-White, 1983).

ASSESSMENT ISSUES

Assessment based on a cross-cultural perspective begins by identifying key differences between partners. First, partners are asked to enumerate differences from their individual perspectives, without consulting with each other. Second, before sharing their respective lists with each other, the partners are asked to indicate whether they experience each difference as toxic, benign, or beneficial to the couple's relationship. To obtain the most useful information on differences, we have found it best to separate the listing and rating tasks, which means not informing the clients that they will be asked to evaluate the differences until after they have identified them.

When the partners have listed and rated their perceived differences, the lists can be compared and discussed. At the outset, it is critical for the therapist to establish that neither partner has the "true tale" and that diverging perspectives are equally valid. Comparing the two lists is likely to reveal meta differences—that is, diverging perceptions about the differences and how they affect the relationship. For example, a marked difference in communication styles may be experienced as benign by one partner and highly toxic by the other.

The next task is to explore the systemic context of the couple's experience of their differences. In some cases, what appear to be "irreconcilable differences" in a given couple may be a cover for one or both partners' not being free to form a partnership outside their family of origin. According to one estimate, in up to 80% of marriages that fail, one or both partners never had permission to succeed in the marriage (Stanton, 1981). In some cases, one or both of the partners have been stabilizing forces in their families of origin. When the adult child leaves to form an intimate partnership, the family of origin may judge the new in-law negatively instead of expressing hurt over perceived abandonment or rejection by the adult child (Friedman, 1982). In other cases, denigration of the new in-law may serve to sustain family-of-origin patterns of closeness, particularly when the spouse confides in the family of origin, rather than the partner, about the trouble in the relationship. Clients frequently are unaware of the systemic context of their experiences of their differences. Thus, the therapist may play a critical role in assessing the systemic context and making the couple aware of it.

When the couple experiences differences as being toxic to their relationship, assessment from a cross-cultural perspective focuses on each partner's cognitive, emotional, and behavioral reactions to these differences. These reactions are interrelated and reciprocally determined (Bandura, 1986).

The cognitive reactions include each person's perceptions of and attributions about the other's unfamiliar behaviors. It is critical to assess: (a) how each partner defines the problem; (b) where each locates the problem; and (c) the meanings each attaches to the behaviors in question. As noted earlier, when asked to define the problem, partners often cast difference as the problem and fail to understand that their difficulty in dealing with difference is more likely to be the culprit causing distress.

Like the definition of the problem, the perceived location of the "problem" can facilitate or interfere with positive change. Typically, couples locate the problem outside themselves: in their partner, in their partner's family of origin, or in their partner's culture—or in some combination of these loci. Whether the problem is located in a person, a family, or a culture, the consequence is the same: the problem is viewed as an unchangeable feature of a system. This perception interferes with communication, understanding, and negotiation, and it typically leads to judgment, further entrenching the couple in their distress. This process can be seen in the following case example of one couple with whom we have worked in cross-cultural couples therapy. (We will use this couple throughout the paper to illustrate various points.)

Pat and Chris were distressed because of their very different strategies for coping with emotional pain. Pat would mask pain by becoming argumentative, legalistic, and openly hostile. In contrast, Chris would become cool and withdrawn, keeping distress concealed. In the initial therapy session, both Pat and Chris located the problem in one another. Moreover, both believed that the other's coping strategy was a personality defect.

The meanings that Pat and Chris attached to one another's behavior also interfered with mutual understanding.

> Chris believed that Pat's behavior demonstrated fear of intimacy. Pat believed that Chris's behavior demonstrated that Chris didn't want or need Pat and that it was only a matter of time before Chris rejected Pat altogether. Both had decided that the respective behaviors were communicating the message, "Stay away; I can't tolerate being close." Both considered the difference in their strategies for coping with pain to be evidence of incompatibility.

In assessing the emotional reactions of each partner to differences, couples therapists should be aware of the intimate link between emotional reactions and cognitive reactions (Hurvitz & Straus, 1991).

> Pat and Chris both felt misunderstood, shut out, untrusted, desperate, and hopeless about finding a solution. These emotional reactions seemed to be a function of each partner's views and interpretations of the other's behaviors as well as the shared belief that the problem resided in the other's intractable personality defects.

The couple's behavioral reactions to perceived differences are related to their cognitive and emotional reactions.

> Chris and Pat's behaviors in the midst of their cross-cultural impasse were as one might have predicted. Experiencing a lack of partner empathy, the couple became further entrenched in familiar coping strategies. Rather than negotiating in the interest of mutual comfort, each exhibited an intensified version of the same behaviors that had proved problematic in the first place. Pat, feeling desperate about making contact with a withdrawing partner, became more controlling and hostile. Chris, motivated by similar feelings but with a different history, withdrew even more. Both partners invested considerable energy in attempting to prove to themselves and to the therapist that their partner's behaviors were to blame for the couple's distress.

Couples who are at a cross-cultural impasse typically either focus on their differences or attempt to deny them.

> Pat and Chris were focusing on their seemingly irreconcilable differences. Difference had become synonymous with incompatibility,

and the consequence was polarization. Each saw the differences that were causing distress as being unchangeable negative features of the other. Pat and Chris became preoccupied with differences, lost sight of common ground, and were well on their way to giving up on the relationship.

Other couples attempt to cope with their cross-cultural conflict by denial. They invest considerable energy in avoiding potential areas of conflict. Whether differences are focused on or denied, the likely result is that essential parts of each individual–which often are differences–will be distorted, discounted, or disregarded.

A final element to be assessed is the origin and function of each partner's cognitive, emotional, and behavioral reactions to differences.

Pat's problematic behaviors were the product of an enmeshed, consuming family of origin. Chris's behaviors were the product of a disengaged, rejecting family of origin. Clearly both sets of behaviors, taken in their original contexts made sense. Pat had learned to fight to get out of a suffocating situation, whereas Chris had learned to hide in order to avoid rejection or ridicule.

INTERVENTION ISSUES

Effective intervention with couples who have difficulty managing their differences involves facilitating the couple's passage through a transition similar to the "cultural transition" required of interracial couples (Falicov & Brudner-White, 1986). The therapist serves as a cross-cultural ambassador between partners' worlds, which requires a thorough understanding of each partner's values and practices and the ways these make sense in historical and systemic context. This understanding enables the therapist to provide translation, interpretation, and mediation to aid the couple's transition.

In the initial session, the therapist explains the cross-cultural perspective to the couple. It is particularly important to emphasize the idea that differences are inevitable and are not problematic in and of themselves. Rather, problems associated with difference often lie in our reactions to the difference itself. Therapists have an opportunity to model this critical perspective by the way they react to differences that couples present. For example, whether a therapist views discrepancies in partners' motivation to work on the relationship as a problem to be solved or as an expected variation will affect the therapist's ability to help the couple (Spiegler, 1991).

Although the focus in cross-cultural couples therapy is on negative experiences of difference, highlighting positive experiences of difference is essential. The therapist should review the differences that the couple perceives as assets or has negotiated successfully. These positive experiences of difference provide inspiration and facilitate working with the differences that are viewed as problematic. Similarly, balancing the focus on differences with a focus on common ground is important. The couple's similarities provide a reservoir of mutual understanding from which partners can draw as they struggle to accept one another's differences.

Cross-cultural couples therapy involves three sequential developmental tasks. First, partners learn to deal with their cognitive, emotional, and behavioral reactivity to their differences. Second, each partner develops some acceptance of the other's differences. Third, the couple co-designs a common culture.

MANAGING PROBLEMATIC REACTIONS TO DIFFERENCE

Many existing interventions can be adapted to help couples manage their problematic reactions to difference. We will present examples of interventions we find especially useful in dealing with partner's cognitive, emotional, and behavioral reactions to difference.

Cognitive Reactions to Difference

One common problematic cognitive reaction to differences concerns the couple's perceived locus of their difficulties. Most couples enter therapy having located the problem in one another. Following Michael White's (1995) example, therapists may attempt to engage the couple in an "externalizing conversation" to relocate the problem away from an individual or a relationship. Thinking they are being sensitive to diversity, some therapists move the problem from the individuals or their relationship to their differences, such as gender (e.g., "He's uninvolved because he's a man"; "She's upset because she's a woman") or ethnicity (e.g., "She's cold because she's a WASP"; "He can't help playing around because he's Latin").

Of course, such attributions are problematic because they are based on reductionistic stereotypes. Moreover, they have the same negative consequences as locating the problem in an individual. They foster a climate of blame and inhibit therapeutic progress by casting the problem as an intractable feature of one's gender or ethnicity. Further, they serve to exonerate the individuals from personal responsibility for their actions, which reduces motivation, disempowers, and engenders helplessness. In sum, locating the problem in the differences interferes with therapeutic progress. It is not enough simply to move the problem *away* from the individuals or their relationship. The problem must be relocated in such a way that a solution is facilitated.

Relocating the problem from the individuals to the *couple's mutual difficulty in dealing with difference* is far more productive. The couple's distress is an indicator, not of personal or background defects, but of transition from living in two diverse personal cultures to living in a co-designed common culture.

Emotional Reactions to Difference

It is not uncommon for couples with marked differences to react to their differences with an almost existential anxiety, which then results in a host of other negative emotions as well as maladaptive cognitions and behaviors. Partners may experience their loved one's unfamiliar behaviors as challenging the validity of their own beliefs and practices, which undermines their self-worth (Gehrie, 1976). A partner may discount, distance, ridicule, or judge the other in a defensive maneuver to ward off anxiety. In other cases, partners respond to differences with feelings of being disconnected, abandoned, or left out. Alternatively, they defend against the pain of alienation with various strategies including hostility, disdain, hatred, and a sense of superiority.

In managing distressing emotional reactions to difference, it is helpful initially to assist partners in exploring their own personal cultures. Most people are unaware of even *having* a personal culture (just as many people naively believe they have no ethnic background because they are "American"). With increased self-understanding and self-acceptance, partner differences become less of a threat and thus emotional reactions to them can be safely examined.

Behavioral Reactions to Difference

Problematic behavioral reactions to difference are best dealt with by providing the client with alternative responses that are both appropriate and fulfill an equivalent function as the problematic behavior (Spiegler & Guevremont, in press). For some reactions, the person may need to learn a new, adaptive response; but in most cases, clients have one or more suitable alternative responses in their repertoire.

Habitual reactions tend to be made "reflexively," with minimal awareness of their being made or of their consequences. Thus, establishing conditions that will reliably prompt the new behavioral response is important.

> Pat's habitual reaction to Chris's withdrawing was to pursue Chris (which exacerbated Chris's withdrawal). Pat was unaware of responding in this manner. The alternative response Pat developed was giving Chris time alone. Pat learned to think "Chris needs space" whenever Chris withdrew, which prompted Pat's new response.

Finally, the new adaptive behavior must be reinforced adequately for it to become a substitute for the old, maladaptive reaction. Reinforcement from one's partner is especially potent because it indicates that the partner is aware of and appreciates the behavioral change. This can be as simple as Chris's thanking Pat for making it easy to take time alone. In addition, self-reinforcement, such as allowing oneself to feel good about making adaptive changes in the interest of the relationship, is necessary because partners generally do not consistently reinforce each other's behaviors. Eventually, the success of the new response will serve as a natural reinforcer that will maintain the behavior.

PROMOTING ACCEPTANCE OF DIFFERENCE

Acceptance as a goal in couples therapy is not a new idea. However, while myriad therapeutic techniques have been developed over the past 100 years for changing how people act, feel, and think, concrete methods for promoting acceptance are lacking.

Two therapeutic strategies that are widely used for various purposes are particularly useful in promoting acceptance in couples. The first involves *personal narratives,* the stories that people construct to explain their life experiences. The second involves cognitive restructuring.

Personal narratives are powerful vehicles for facilitating acceptance of differences. Imbedded in personal narratives are the guiding personal myths that people have developed to explain significant life events. The personal myths are "supernatural explanations which legitimize, justify, and preserve personal values, behaviors, norms and mores" (Bagarozzi & Anderson, 1989). They are essential for a sense of coherence in one's life.

Besides providing explanations of past experiences, personal myths serve as templates from which expectations of the future are generated.

Listening deeply to another's narrative provides a context within which partners begin to make sense of beliefs and practices that previously seemed offensive or intolerable.

> Pat became enraged when Chris would withdraw in the midst of a conflict. In Pat's personal culture, withdrawal was an act of disloyalty and abandonment. Pat therefore interpreted Chris's behavior as an indication that Chris really did not want to be in the relationship. To Chris, however, withdrawal was an effective mechanism learned for coping with family-of-origin conflicts that tended to end in "alcoholic meltdowns" involving painful verbal abuse. As Pat came to understand this from hearing Chris's narrative, Pat was able to stop personalizing Chris's withdrawal and appreciate its survival value for Chris.

Having taken in and learned to "hold" one another's narratives, partners begin to move from judgment to acceptance. Genuine listening yields the appreciation of and respect for differences that make it possible to move beyond the stalemate over whose personal culture is more valid or worthy.

A second strategy for promoting acceptance is *cognitive restructuring,* the process of identifying dysfunctional cognitions (thoughts, beliefs) and substituting more functional cognitions for them (Spiegler & Guevremont, 1993). In cross-cultural couples therapy, partners are asked to cognitively reconstrue (i.e., view differently) how they evaluate the other's differences. Minimally, the goal of cognitive restructuring is to make the differences less negative and more palatable (cf. Ellis, 1993). For example, a difference initially seen as "intolerable" might be reconstrued as "annoying."

Ideally, the goal of cognitive restructuring is to have partners come to evaluate differences as positive (Jacobson, 1992). To achieve this more ambitious goal, the therapist guides the couple in discovering that all undesirable behaviors are the flip side of desirable behaviors. Indeed, the flip side of the "toxic" differences often turn out to be the very behaviors that made the partner attractive in the first place (e.g., smothering versus attentive).

We use an exercise to help couples discover this new perspective. We ask each partner to compile a written list of the other partner's "undesirable" behaviors. Not surprisingly, couples in distress easily and enthusiastically complete this task. Then, we ask each partner to make a list of the other's "desirable" behaviors. As might be expected, couples often find this task difficult, especially if they are focusing on their partner's current behaviors. Suggesting the inclusion of behaviors from a more satisfying time in their relationship (e.g., during courtship) generally leads to a larger list. We prefer not to make this suggestion immediately, however, in the hope that each partner will generate at least some present desirable behaviors.

The lists are compared to discover desirable behaviors that are the flip side of the undesirable behaviors, such as: "thoughtful" and "moody"; "careful" and "picky"; and "creative" and "scatterbrained" (Spiegler & Guevremont, 1993). The exercise provides couples with an understanding that all behaviors can be evaluated either as desirable or as undesirable. In one sense, you can't have one without the other (or at least the potential for the other). Cognitive restructuring exercises teach a generalizable skill for coping with the inevitable differences that continue to surface throughout a couple relationship.

Earlier we said that change sometimes is not a realistic or even appropriate goal for dealing with differences in intimate relationships. Actually, both understanding of personal narratives and cognitive restructuring involve change (e.g., Baucom & Epstein, 1991; Snyder & Wills, 1991). However, the change is one of perspectives rather than overt behavior. Moreover, the change is required of each partner, rather than being something one partner requires of the other.

HELPING COUPLES CO-CONSTRUCT A COMMON CULTURE

Once couples have learned to manage their own reactivity toward one another's differences and have begun to appreciate and accept the differences, they are ready to begin co-constructing a common couple culture. We employ three strategies to assist couples in forging a common culture: (1) negotiating points of difference; (2) designing and carrying out rituals to validate the newly co-constructed common culture; and (3) creating a united front to protect the couple culture from destructive elements beyond the couple relationship.

Negotiating points of difference involves the delicate and respectful process of distinguishing the beliefs and practices that are essential to each individual, and therefore non-negotiable, from those that are alterable without subverting the individual's stability. In the end, the co-designed culture will include some practices that have been altered and some that remain unchanged.

There was something essential to Pat about being a "pack rat," whereas Chris preferred to throw out anything not currently in use. Chris had reacted to Pat's behavior with anger, feeling that Pat was selfishly imposing chaos on the household. During therapy, Chris came to understand that saving things made Pat feel secure, and Chris was able to accept Pat's behavior. In contrast, Pat also had a long-standing habit of being late, which conflicted with Chris's valuing being punctual. Punctuality was essential to Chris's well being, as it symbolized predictability in what had been a chaotic family of origin. Since, for Pat, being late was related only to time management and was not essential to a sense of well being, this difference was negotiable. In these and numerous other areas of difference, Pat and Chris learned to accept non-negotiable behaviors and agreed to change negotiable behaviors in order to accommodate one another's needs.

Rituals can be used to facilitate cultural transition by validating diverging individual positions and, at the same time, creating consensus (Imber-Black, Roberts, & Whiting, 1988).

Chris preferred to let conflicts "blow over," whereas Pat felt strongly about the importance of talking disagreements through, for hours if necessary, until some resolution could be reached. A variation of the Milan team's odd days/even days prescription proved useful (Selvini Palazzoli, Boscolo, Cecchin, & Prata, 1978). For a two week period, Chris and Pat agreed to try out three-day cycles in which they would let problems "blow over" on the first day, talk them through to resolution on the second day, and discuss problems for a maximum of 20 minutes at a predetermined time on the third day. This ritual generated empathy by providing a structure that allowed each partner to "try on," without having to commit to change, the other's preferred strategy for dealing with conflict. Toward the end of the second week, the couple reached a consensus that the third-day alternative would work for both of them.

Rituals that serve to mark the transition from the former disparate personal cultures to the newly co-constructed couple culture should incorporate a combination of the personal symbolism of each partner and symbolism that represents the couple's common culture. One such ritual involves each partner choosing a separate symbol of his or her difficulty dealing with a particular difference, and the couple selecting a common symbol of acceptance of the difference. The couple then designs a ritual in which the symbols of problematic reactions to the difference are transformed and the symbol of acceptance of the difference is given a prominent place in their lives.

> Chris and Pat created a ritual that involved symbols for their difficulty with disparate styles of conflict resolution and a symbol for their acceptance of their differences. Chris chose a large paper bag to hide under, and Pat chose a cardboard megaphone to accentuate points during endless discussions. The couple decided to burn the bag and megaphone and sprinkle the ashes on their garden. Then the couple bought a decorative hour glass which they used to time their scheduled conflict resolution sessions.

Newly formed couple cultures may disrupt the balance of existing larger relationship systems (such as family of origin and friends) in which the couple system is embedded. Accordingly, a couple may have to deal with resistance from the larger systems as the members of the systems adapt to the new couple culture. Rituals can help define the couple's common cultural code to the outside world and prevent its being subverted.

> When Pat and Chris visited Pat's highly enmeshed family, Pat's parents frequently engaged in extended conversations with their child as though Chris were not there. This pattern became increasingly intolerable to the couple because the cohesion that they had worked so hard to achieve seemed to dissolve in the presence of Pat's family of origin. Hence, the couple designed a ritual in which each time the sequence began, Pat would turn and seek Chris's counsel on the matter under discussion. Without engaging in confrontation, the couple made it clear to Pat's parents that they were a team and could not be split in the interest of perpetuating the exclusive closeness that had characterized Pat's pre-partnership parent-child relationship.

CONCLUSION

We believe that it is useful to view every couple as a cross-cultural relationship. This perspective provides direction for working with the inevitable differences couples experience. The cross-cultural perspective focuses on partners' maladaptive reactions to differences, rather than the differences themselves, as targets for intervention. The goal of cross-cultural couples therapy is for the couple to come to accept differences and to co-construct a common couple culture.

REFERENCES

Atkinson, D. R., & Hackett, G. (1995). *Counseling diverse populations.* Dubuque, IA: William C. Brown.

Atkinson, D. R., Morten, G. & Sue, D. W. (1989). *Counseling American minorities: A cross-cultural perspective* (3rd ed.). Dubuque, IA: William C. Brown.

Axelson, J. A. (1993). *Counseling and development in a multicultural society.* Pacific Grove, CA: Brooks/Cole.

Bagarozzi, D. A., & Anderson, S. A. (1989). *Personal, marital, and family myths: Theoretical formulations and clinical strategies.* New York: Norton.

Bandura, A. (1986). *Social foundations of thought and action: A social cognitive theory.* Englewood Cliffs, NJ: Prentice-Hall.

Baucom, D. H., & Epstein, N. (1991). Will the real cognitive-behavioral marital therapy please stand up? *Journal of Family Psychology, 4,* 394-401.

Braverman, L. (1995, July/August). Chasing rainbows. *The Family Therapy Networker, 17,* 36-41, 69-71.

Ellis, A. (1993). Fundamentals of rational-emotive therapy for the 1990's. In W. Dryden & L. K. Hill (Eds.), *Innovations in rational-emotive therapy* (pp. 1-32). Newbury Park, CA: Sage Publications.

Falicov, C. J., & Brudner-White, L. (1983). The shifting family triangle: The issue of cultural and contextual relativity. In C.J. Falicov (ed.), *Cultural perspectives in family therapy.* Rockville, MD: Aspen Systems.

Friedman, E. (1982). The myth of the shiksa. In M. McGoldrick, J. K. Pearce, & J. Giordano (Eds.), *Ethnicity and family therapy.* New York: Guilford Press.

Gehrie, M. (1976). Aspects of dynamics of prejudice. *Annual of Review of Psychoanalysis, 4,* 423-446.

Hurvitz, N., & Straus, R. A. (1991). *Marriage and family therapy: A sociocognitive approach.* New York: The Haworth Press, Inc.

Imber-Black, E., Roberts, J., & Whiting, R. (Eds.). (1988). *Rituals in families and family therapy.* New York: Norton.

Jacobson, N. S. (1992). Behavioral couple therapy: A new beginning. *Behavior Therapy, 23,* 493-506.

Liebert, R. M., & Spiegler, M. D. (1994). *Personality: Strategies and issues* (7th ed.). Pacific Grove, CA: Brooks/Cole.

Pinderhughes, E. (1989). *Understanding race, ethnicity, and power: The key to efficacy in clinical practice.* New York: Free Press.

Reiss, D. (1976). *Family systems in America.* Hinsdale, IL: Dryden Press.

Selvini Palazzoli, M., Boscolo, L., Cecchin, G., & Prata, G. (1978). A ritualized prescription in family therapy: Odd days and even days. *Journal of Marital and Family Therapy, 10,* 253-271.

Shaver, P., & Hazan, C., & Bradshaw, D. (1988). Love as attachment: The integration of three behavioral systems. In R. J. Sternberg & M. L. Barnes (Eds.), *The psychology of love.* New Haven: Yale University Press.

Snyder, D. K., & Wills, R. M. (1991). Facilitating change in marital therapy and research. *Journal of Family Psychology, 4,* 426-435.

Spiegler, M. D. (1991). Satir's formula for therapeutic endurance: The wonderful human being myth. *Journal of Couples Therapy, 2,* 165-167.

Spiegler, M. D., & Guevremont, D. C. (1993). *Contemporary behavior therapy* (2nd ed.). Pacific Grove, CA: Brooks/Cole.

Spiegler, M. D., & Guevremont, D. C. (in press). *Contemporary behavior therapy* (3rd ed.). Pacific Grove, CA: Brooks/Cole.

Stanton, M.D. (1981). Marital therapy from a structural/strategic viewpoint. In G. P. Sholevar (Ed.). *The handbook of marriage and marital therapy.* Jamaica, NY: S. P. Medical and Scientific Books.

White, M. (1995). *Re-authoring lives: Interviews and essays.* Adelaide, South Australia: Delwich Centre Publications.

Winch, R. (1955). The theory of complementary needs in mate selection: Final results on the test of the general hypothesis. *American Sociological Review, 20,* 553-555.

Index

Abandonment, fear of, 15,63
Ability, power as, 32
Absent partners
    therapists' handling of, 20-21
    in violence counseling, 75-76
Absorption, fear of, 15
Abuse
    child, 78
    spousal, 49-81. *See also* Violence
Ackerman Institute spousal abuse
    model, 52
ACOAs, 5,22,92,93
Adapted Child concept, 60f
Addiction, 13-14,62
    spousal abuse as, 67
Addictive coping, 62-63
Adultery, 21-23,39-40
"Alcoholic meltdowns," 93
Alcoholism, 5. *See also* ACOAs
American Family Therapy
    Association, 52
Analogous experience technique, 18
Analytic/systemic approach
    integration, 9-25
    case example, 21-24
    couple dynamics in intimacy
        issues, 12-16
    forms of resistance and, 12-13
    individual dynamics in couple
        resistance, 10-12
    rationale for, 10-14
    techniques and tactics, 16-21.
        See also Therapeutic
        techniques
Anger, 68. *See also* Violence
    generation versus feeling of, 55
Anxiety, 18
    in violent relationships, 63

Approach/withdraw couple dance,
    30-31
Arguments, "silly," 30
Arousal, emotional, 59-61,61f
Assessment
    of couple dynamics, 19
    of cross-cultural differences,
        85-89,87-89
    instruments for, 34-35
    of power struggles, 33-36
Assumptive values, 14-15
Astor, Martin, 9-25,24n
Attitudes
    about marriage, 10
    toward change, 2,5-6
Attunement, symbiotic, 14
Avanta Process Community Meeting
    III, 1-7

Background issues, 14-15
Bader-Pearson Couple Diagnostic
    Questionnaire, 34,35-36
Banana/broken hip analogy, 3-4
Banmen, John, 1-7
Battering, 49-81. *See also* Violence
Behavior(s)
    demands for change in, 15
    double-level, 5
    male versus female in workplace,
        44-45
    personality as explanation of,
        54-55
    reciprocal reinforcement of, 15
    as trigger for violence, 61-62
    written lists of, 93-94
Behavioral effects, of cycle of
    violence, 71-73

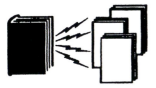

Haworth
DOCUMENT DELIVERY
SERVICE

This valuable service provides a single-article order form for any article from a Haworth journal.

- *Time Saving:* No running around from library to library to find a specific article.
- *Cost Effective:* All costs are kept down to a minimum.
- *Fast Delivery:* Choose from several options, including same-day FAX.
- *No Copyright Hassles:* You will be supplied by the original publisher.
- *Easy Payment:* Choose from several easy payment methods.

Open Accounts Welcome for ...
- Library Interlibrary Loan Departments
- Library Network/Consortia Wishing to Provide Single-Article Services
- Indexing/Abstracting Services with Single Article Provision Services
- Document Provision Brokers and Freelance Information Service Providers

---

MAIL or *FAX* THIS ENTIRE ORDER FORM TO:

Haworth Document Delivery Service
The Haworth Press, Inc.
10 Alice Street
Binghamton, NY 13904-1580

or FAX: 1-800-895-0582
or CALL: 1-800-342-9678
9am-5pm EST

PLEASE SEND ME PHOTOCOPIES OF THE FOLLOWING SINGLE ARTICLES:

1) Journal Title: _____

   Vol/Issue/Year: _____ Starting & Ending Pages: _____

Article Title: _____

_____

2) Journal Title: _____

   Vol/Issue/Year: _____ Starting & Ending Pages: _____

Article Title: _____

_____

3) Journal Title: _____

   Vol/Issue/Year: _____ Starting & Ending Pages: _____

Article Title: _____

_____

4) Journal Title: _____

   Vol/Issue/Year: _____ Starting & Ending Pages: _____

Article Title: _____

(See other side for Costs and Payment Information)

COSTS: Please figure your cost to order quality copies of an article.

1. Set-up charge per article: $8.00

    ($8.00 × number of separate articles)   _____

2. Photocopying charge for each article:

    1-10 pages: $1.00   _____

    11-19 pages: $3.00   _____

    20-29 pages: $5.00   _____

    30+ pages: $2.00/10 pages   _____

3. Flexicover (optional): $2.00/article   _____

4. Postage & Handling: US: $1.00 for the first article/

    $.50 each additional article   _____

    Federal Express: $25.00   _____

    Outside US: $2.00 for first article/

    $.50 each additional article   _____

5. Same-day FAX service: $.35 per page   _____

                GRAND TOTAL: _____

METHOD OF PAYMENT: (please check one)

❑ Check enclosed   ❑ Please ship and bill. PO # _____

    (sorry we can ship and bill to bookstores only! All others must pre-pay)

❑ Charge to my credit card: ❑ Visa; ❑ MasterCard; ❑ Discover;

               ❑ American Express;

Account Number: _____ Expiration date: _____

Signature: ✗_____

Name: _____ Institution: _____

Address: _____

_____

City: _____ State: _____ Zip: _____

Phone Number: _____ FAX Number: _____

MAIL or *FAX* THIS ENTIRE ORDER FORM TO:

Haworth Document Delivery Service   **or FAX:** 1-800-895-0582
The Haworth Press, Inc.   **or CALL:** 1-800-342-9678
10 Alice Street   9am-5pm EST)
Binghamton, NY 13904-1580